"The greatest book you will ever read
is the one you write."
– Doreen Rivera

Doreen Rivera's The Bodyful Mind
...A Process of Evolution®

THE BODY has an intelligence, energy in motion, an internal communication that is constant, though we may have very little recognition as to the varied depth of that communication.

The purpose of this journal is to build a deeper relationship to the communications that our body provides in the forms of thoughts, feelings, and sensations. These sensations are and have been continuously recorded in the cells of our bodies. All of these recordings are activated through the physical and emotional movements that occur in daily life. This fact is what we consciously acknowledge and explore in The Bodyful Mind Process®. Whether you're conscious of the recordings or not, there is a stream of information that flows forth from the cells of the physical body continuously, and all of it has great value.

The Bodyful Mind Process® is a journey inward that will provide you with a deeper connection to your inner world. In this journal, note every thought, every feeling, everything you hear in your head as you do a movement. Rather than dismiss the feelings or try to quiet your mind, write all of it down, just exactly as it came to you, especially the thoughts and feelings you want to dismiss.

Then consider what part of the body you were exercising when these thoughts, feelings, etc. came up. Let's say, for example, you were working your arms and your shoulders became tense. Use the figure at the bottom of the pages that follow to indicate what area of the body you were working when these thoughts and feelings occurred. Check the body map on the preceding page. You will discover that shoulders are about responsibility, and tension indicates a holding on. Explore and consider what you are holding onto in terms of your belief about your responsibilities. This is an example of how to use the journal and the body map. Everything you learn from your body has value.

As you write, continue to explore the information that your body is teaching you. You may become aware of patterns held in particular areas of the body that hold certain experience. Use the body map to piece together a deeper understanding about the story your body holds as truth vs. what your mind has been trained to believe.

Be willing, be open, stay curious and allow for a deeper experience of yourself to emerge from within.

Enjoy the journey!

Doreen Rivera

♥ THE BASIC BODYFUL MIND BODYMAP® ♥

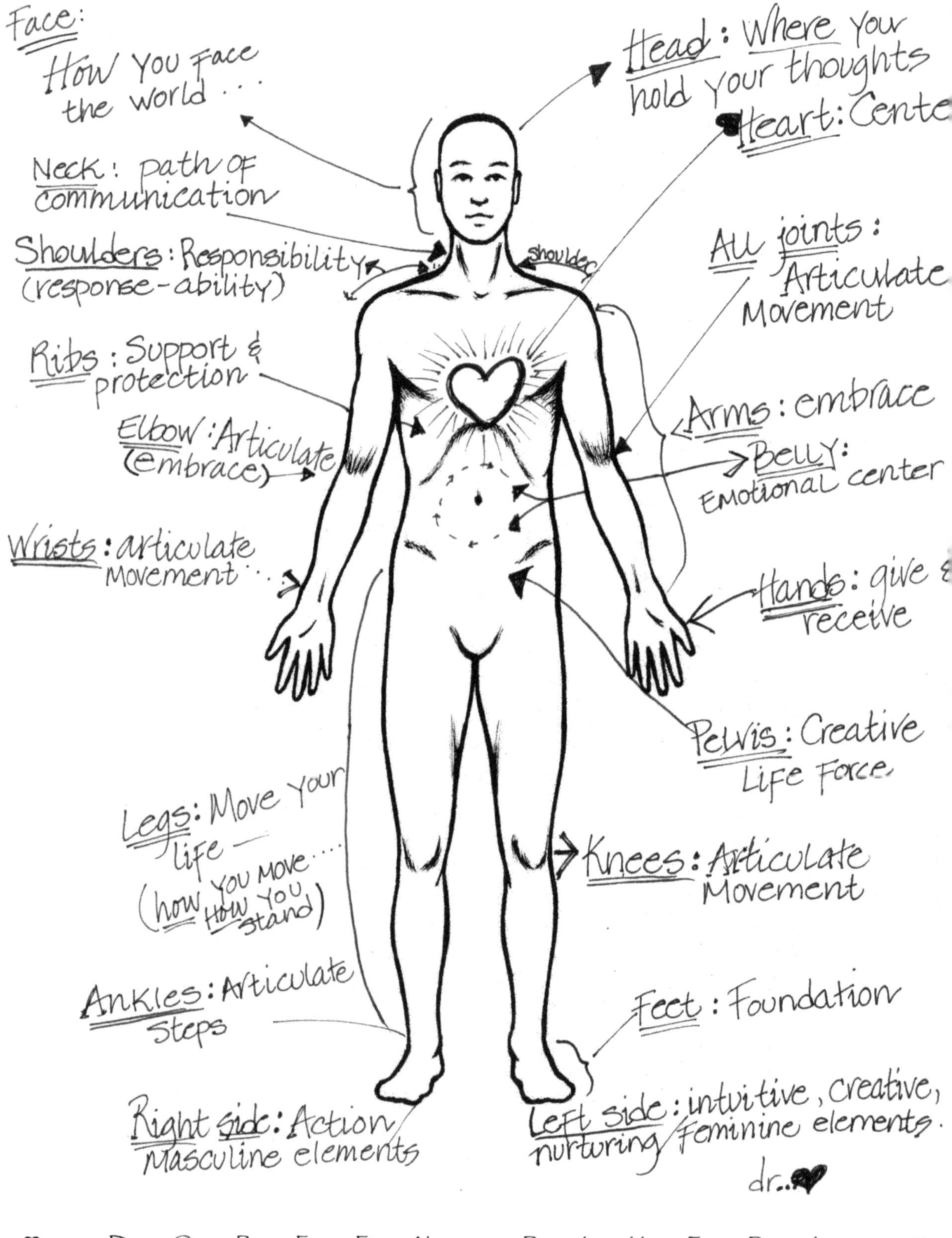

♥ DOREEN RIVERA ♥

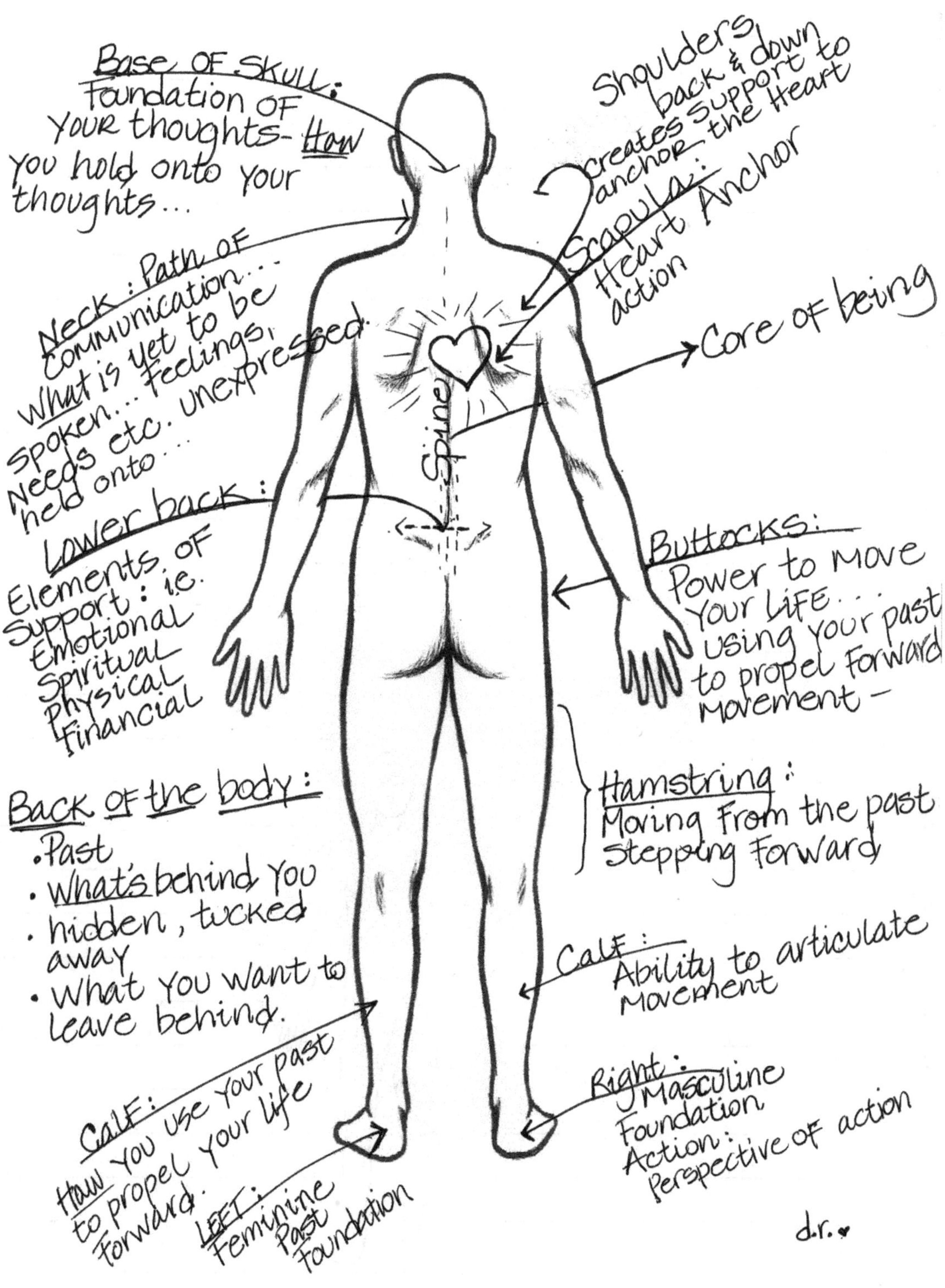
Base of Skull: Foundation of your thoughts- How you hold onto your thoughts...
Shoulders back & down creates support to anchor the Heart
Scapula: Heart Anchor action
Neck: Path of Communication... What is yet to be spoken... feelings, needs etc. unexpressed held onto...
Core of being
Spine
Lower back: Elements of Support: i.e. Emotional Spiritual Physical Financial
Buttocks: Power to move your life... using your past to propel forward movement -
Back of the body:
• Past
• What's behind you
• hidden, tucked away
• What you want to leave behind.
Hamstring: Moving from the past Stepping forward
Calf: Ability to articulate movement
Calf: How you use your past to propel your life forward.
Right: Masculine Foundation Action: Perspective of action
Left: Feminine Past Foundation
d.r.♥

ASK YOURSELF QUESTIONS ♥ ASK YOURSELF QUESTIONS

ASK YOURSELF QUESTIONS ♥ ASK YOURSELF QUESTIONS

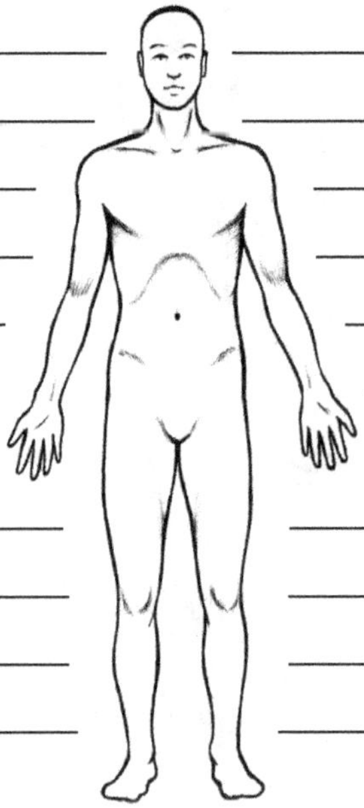

ASK YOURSELF QUESTIONS ♥ ASK YOURSELF QUESTIONS

ASK YOURSELF QUESTIONS ♥ ASK YOURSELF QUESTIONS ♥

ASK YOURSELF QUESTIONS ♥ ASK YOURSELF QUESTIONS

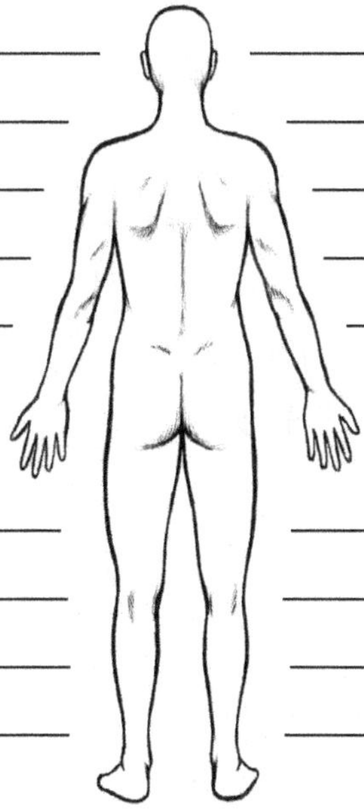

ASK YOURSELF QUESTIONS ♥ ASK YOURSELF QUESTIONS ♥

SEEK THE ANSWER WITHIN ♥ SEEK THE ANSWER WITHIN

SEEK THE ANSWER WITHIN ♥ SEEK THE ANSWER WITHIN

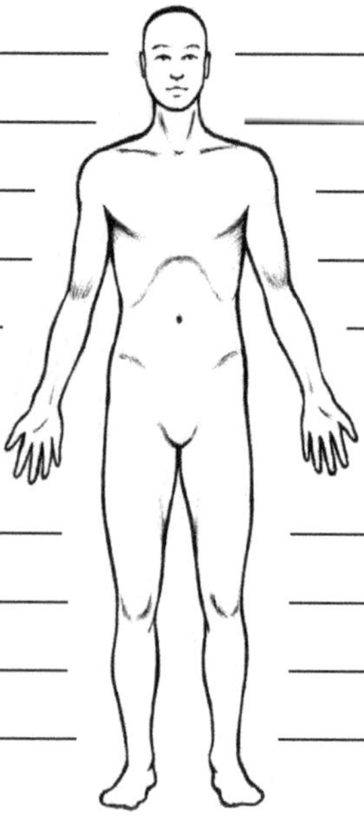

SEEK THE ANSWER WITHIN ♥ SEEK THE ANSWER WITHIN

SEEK THE ANSWER WITHIN ♥ SEEK THE ANSWER WITHIN ♥

SEEK THE ANSWER WITHIN ♥ SEEK THE ANSWER WITHIN

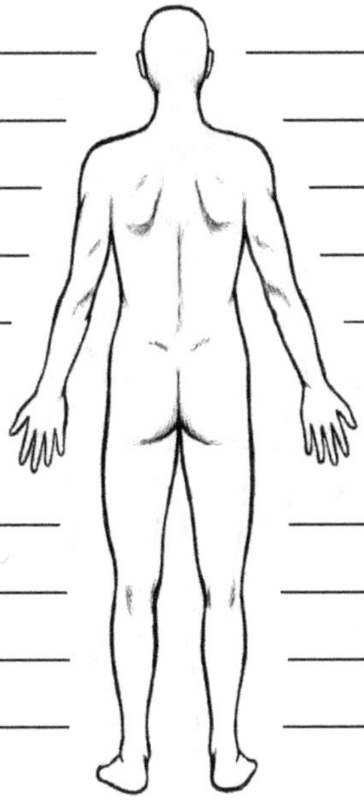

SEEK THE ANSWER WITHIN ♥ SEEK THE ANSWER WITHIN ♥

FEET: FOUNDATION ❤ FEET: FOUNDATION ❤ FEET: FOUNDATION

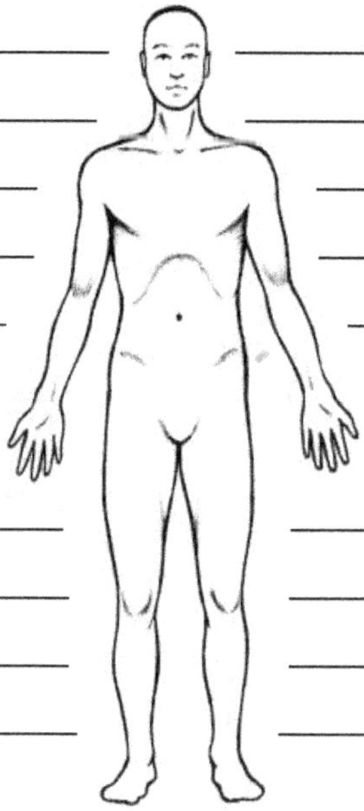

FEET: FOUNDATION ♥ FEET: FOUNDATION ♥ FEET: FOUNDATION

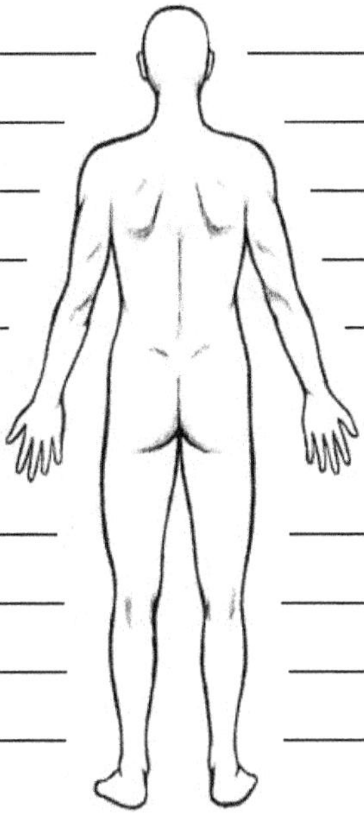

FEET: FOUNDATION ♥ FEET: FOUNDATION ♥

BE CURIOUS ♥ BE CURIOUS

BE CURIOUS ♥ BE CURIOUS ♥ BE CURIOUS

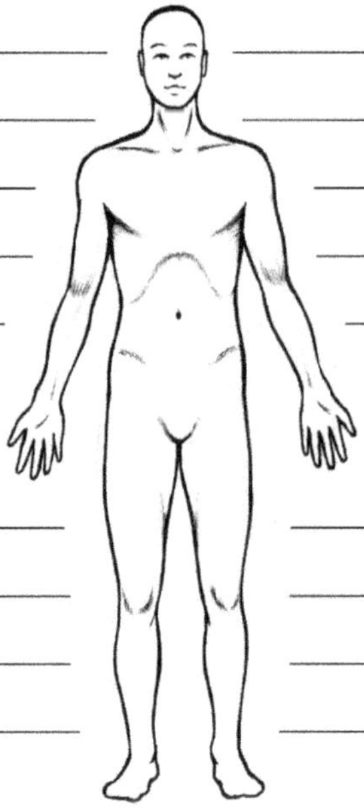

BE CURIOUS ♥ BE CURIOUS

BE CURIOUS ❤ BE CURIOUS ❤

BE CURIOUS ❤ BE CURIOUS ❤ BE CURIOUS

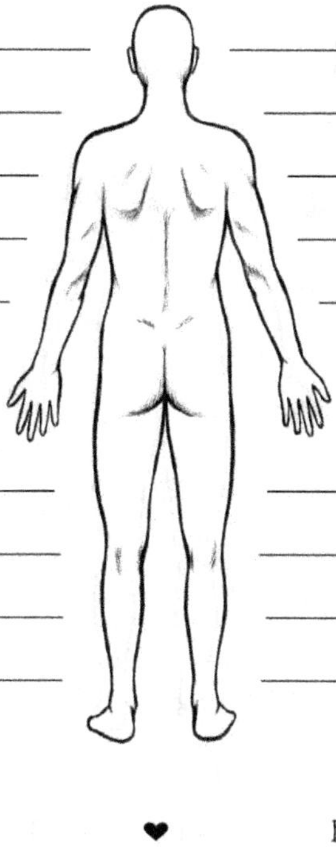

BE CURIOUS ❤ BE CURIOUS ❤

JOINTS: ARTICULATE MOVEMENT • JOINTS: ARTICULATE MOVEMENT

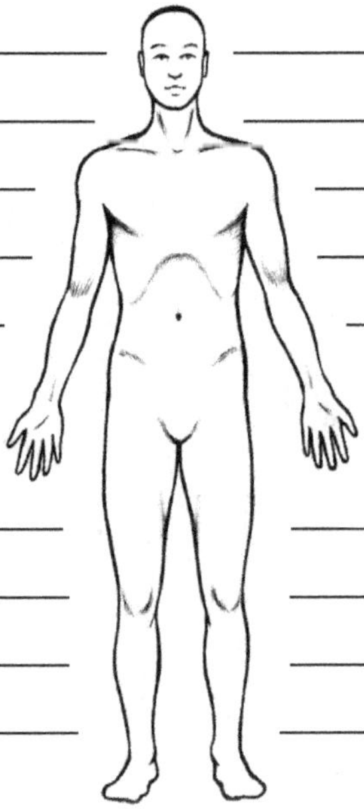

JOINTS: ARTICULATE MOVEMENT

JOINTS: ARTICULATE MOVEMENT

JOINTS: ARTICULATE MOVEMENT

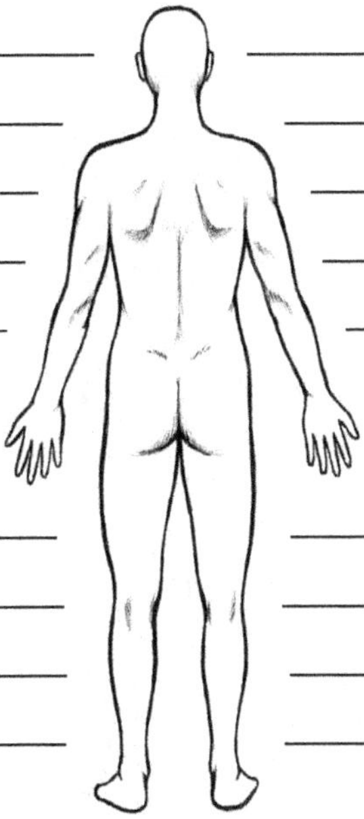

MOVE INTO YOURSELF ♥ MOVE INTO YOURSELF

MOVE INTO YOURSELF ♥ MOVE INTO YOURSELF ♥ MOVE INTO YOURSELF

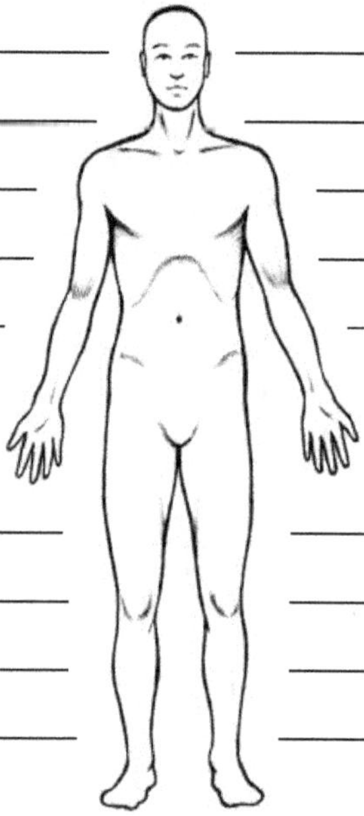

MOVE INTO YOURSELF ♥ MOVE INTO YOURSELF

MOVE INTO YOURSELF ♥ MOVE INTO YOURSELF ♥

MOVE INTO YOURSELF ♥ MOVE INTO YOURSELF ♥ MOVE INTO YOURSELF

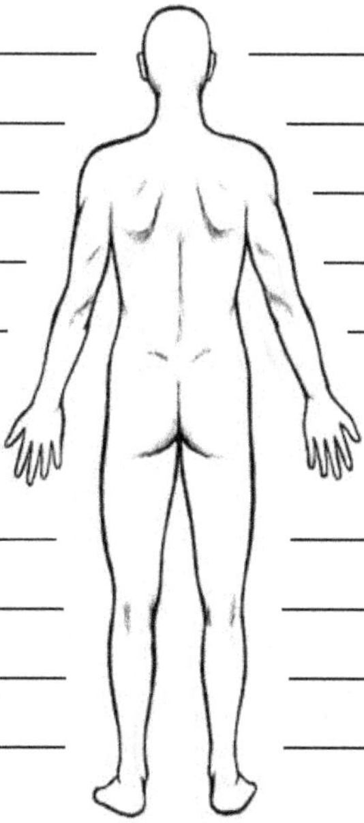

MOVE INTO YOURSELF ♥ MOVE INTO YOURSELF ♥

LEGS: HOW YOU STAND & MOVE ♥ LEGS: HOW YOU STAND & MOVE

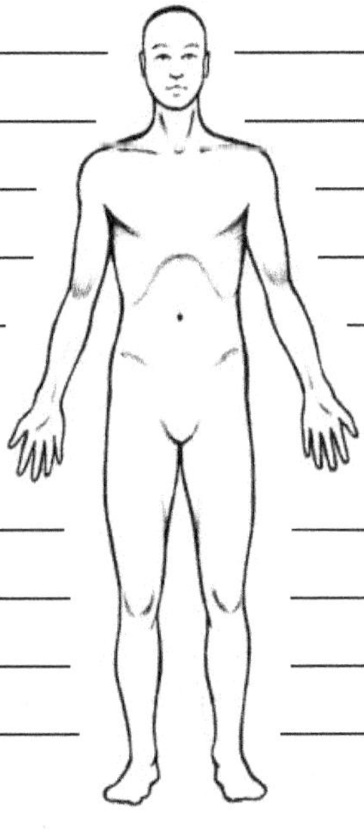

LEGS: HOW YOU STAND & MOVE ♥ LEGS: HOW YOU STAND & MOVE

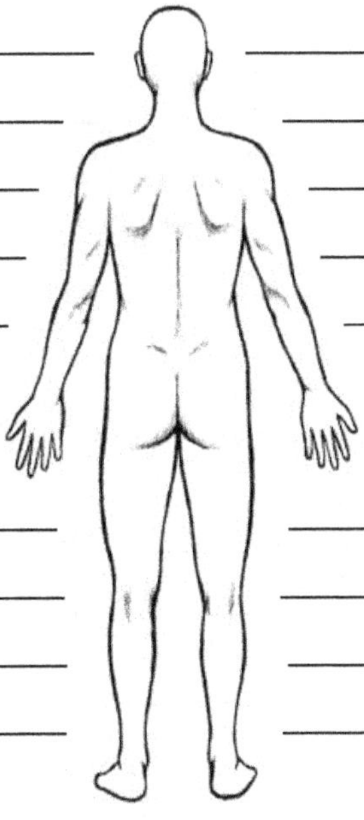

FOLLOW THE FEELINGS ♥ FOLLOW THE FEELINGS

FOLLOW THE FEELINGS ♥ FOLLOW THE FEELINGS

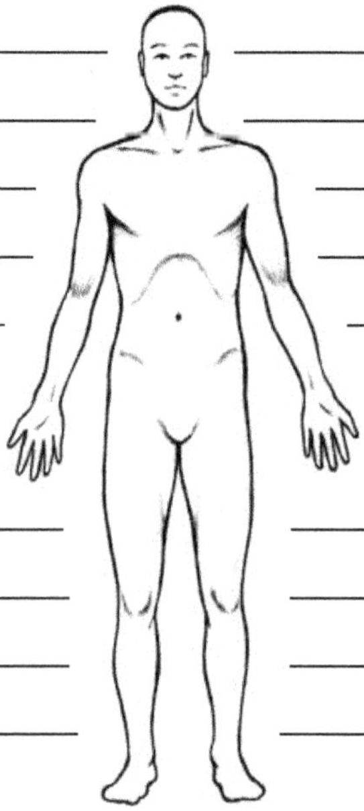

FOLLOW THE FEELINGS ♥ FOLLOW THE FEELINGS

FOLLOW THE FEELINGS ♥ FOLLOW THE FEELINGS

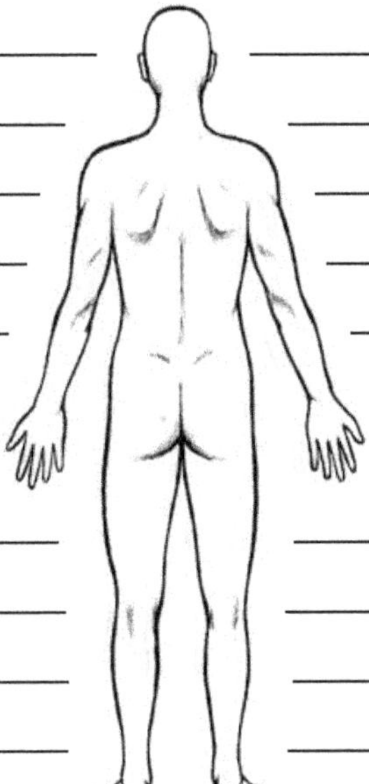

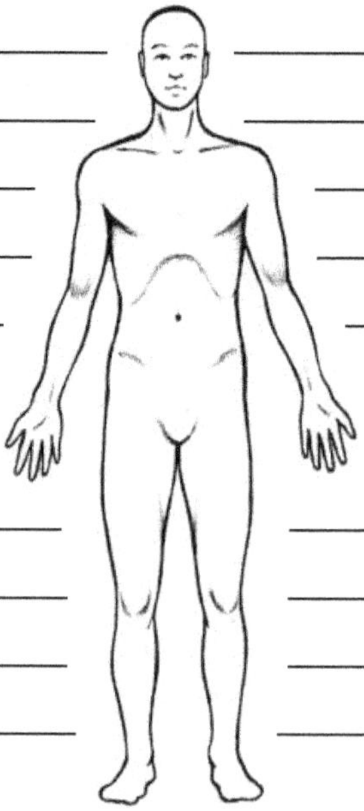

PELVIS: CREATIVE LIFE FORCE ♥ PELVIS: CREATIVE LIFE FORCE

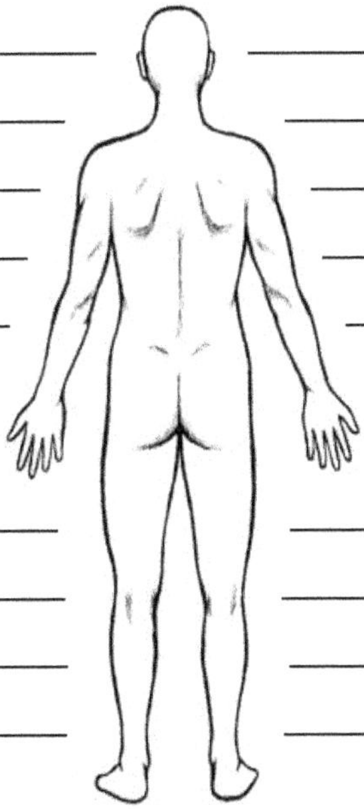

EXPLORE THE EXPERIENCE EXPLORE THE EXPERIENCE

EXPLORE THE EXPERIENCE
EXPLORE THE EXPERIENCE

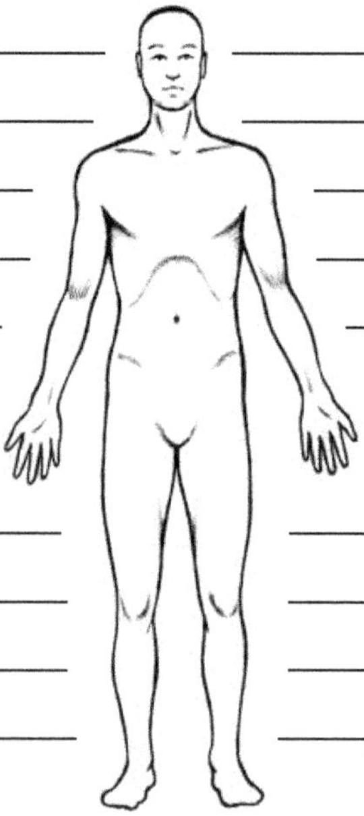

EXPLORE THE EXPERIENCE EXPLORE THE EXPERIENCE

EXPLORE THE EXPERIENCE ♥ EXPLORE THE EXPERIENCE

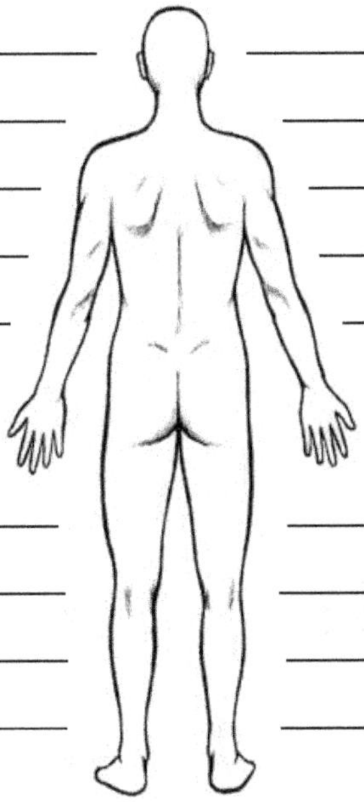

BELLY: EMOTIONAL CENTER ♥ BELLY: EMOTIONAL CENTER ♥ BELLY: EMOTIONAL CENTER

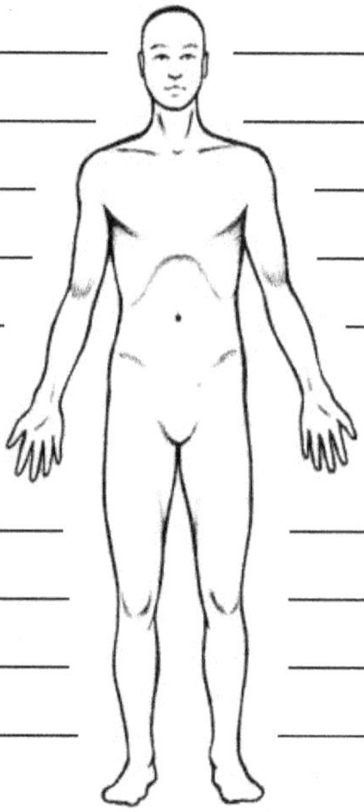

BELLY: EMOTIONAL CENTER ♥ BELLY: EMOTIONAL CENTER ♥ BELLY: EMOTIONAL CENTER

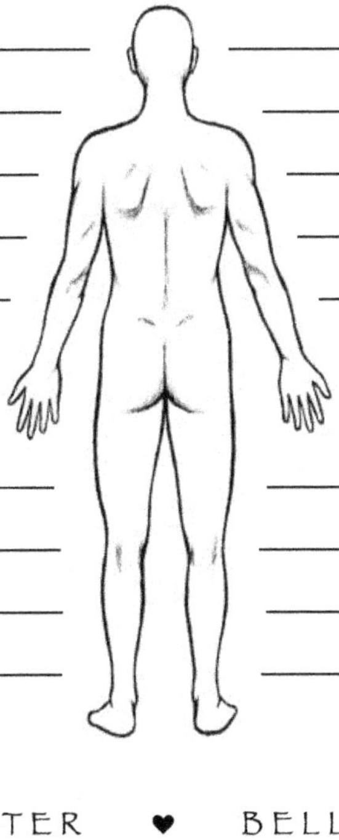

BELLY: EMOTIONAL CENTER ♥ BELLY: EMOTIONAL CENTER ♥

ANSWER TO YOUR FEELINGS ♥ ANSWER TO YOUR FEELINGS

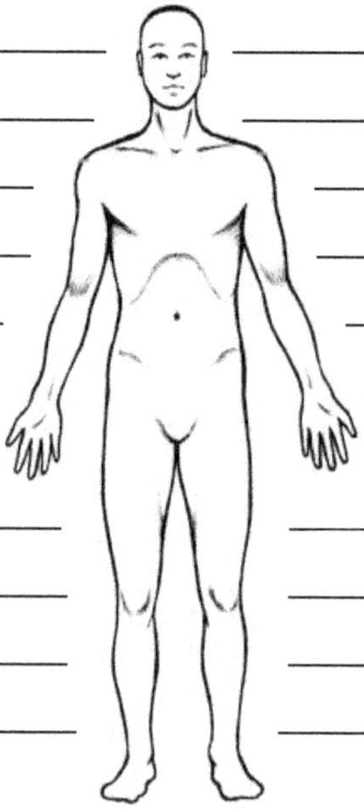

ANSWER TO YOUR FEELINGS ♥ ANSWER TO YOUR FEELINGS
ANSWER TO YOUR FEELINGS ♥ ANSWER TO YOUR FEELINGS

ANSWER TO YOUR FEELINGS ♥ ANSWER TO YOUR FEELINGS

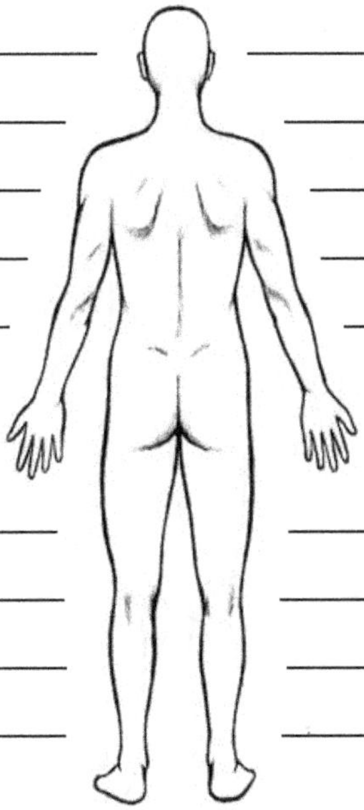

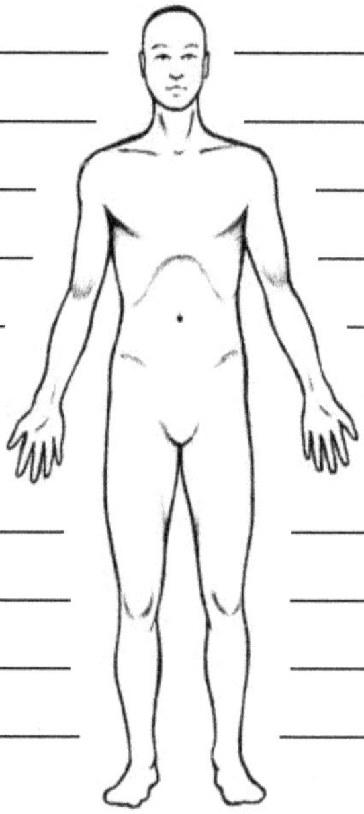

CHEST: HEART CENTER ♥ CHEST: HEART CENTER ♥ CHEST: HEART CENTER

CHEST: HEART CENTER ♥ CHEST: HEART CENTER

CHEST: HEART CENTER ❤ CHEST: HEART CENTER ❤ CHEST: HEART CENTER

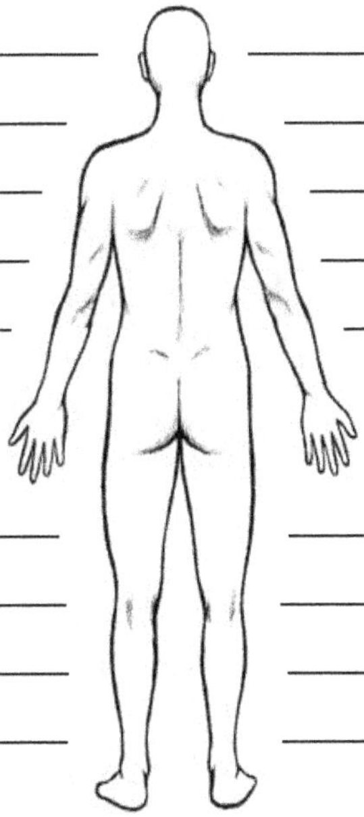

LEAD WITH YOUR HEART ♥ LEAD WITH YOUR HEART

LEAD WITH YOUR HEART ♥ LEAD WITH YOUR HEART

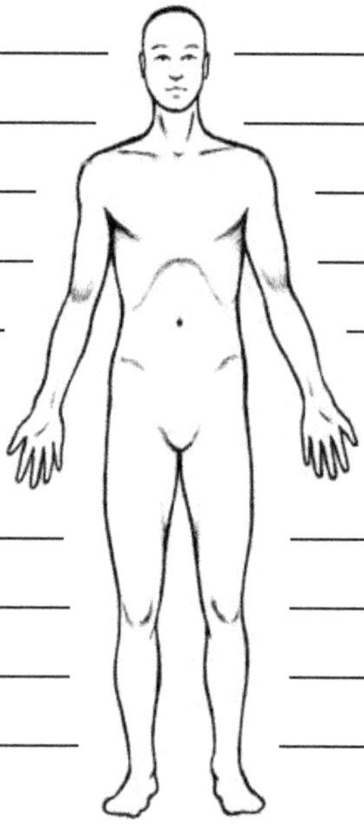

LEAD WITH YOUR HEART ♥ LEAD WITH YOUR HEART

LEAD WITH YOUR HEART ♥ LEAD WITH YOUR HEART ♥

LEAD WITH YOUR HEART ♥ LEAD WITH YOUR HEART

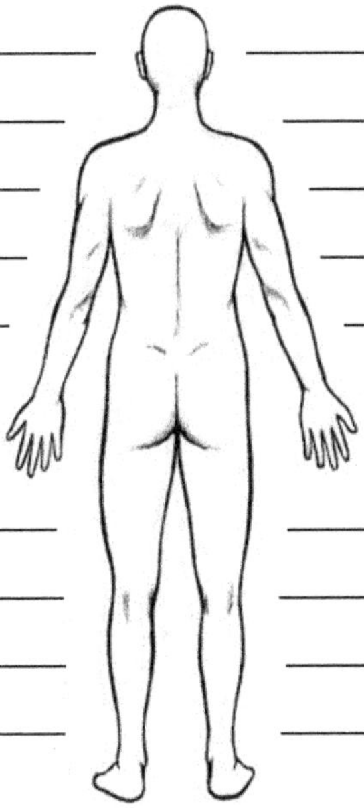

LEAD WITH YOUR HEART ♥ LEAD WITH YOUR HEART ♥

RIBS: HEART SUPPORT

RIBS: HEART SUPPORT
RIBS: HEART SUPPORT
RIBS: HEART SUPPORT

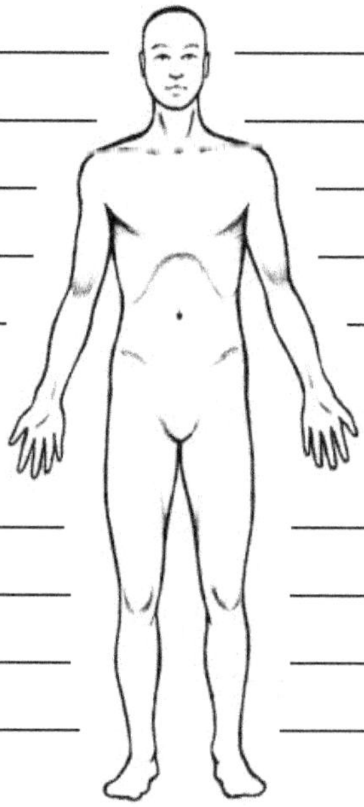

RIBS: HEART SUPPORT
RIBS: HEART SUPPORT

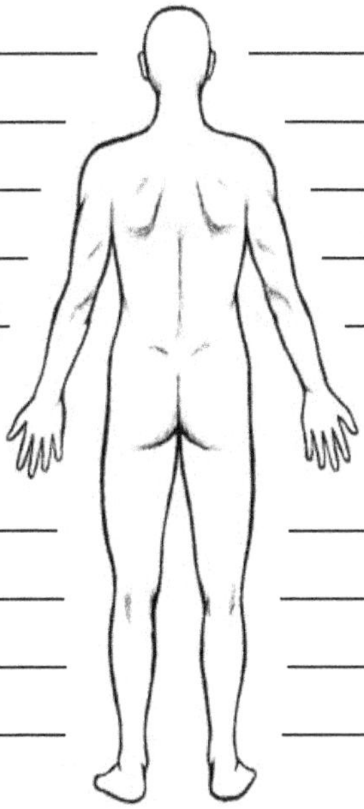

RIBS: HEART SUPPORT ♥ RIBS: HEART SUPPORT ♥ RIBS: HEART SUPPORT

TRUST YOUR HEART ♥ TRUST YOUR HEART

TRUST YOUR HEART ♥ TRUST YOUR HEART ♥ TRUST YOUR HEART

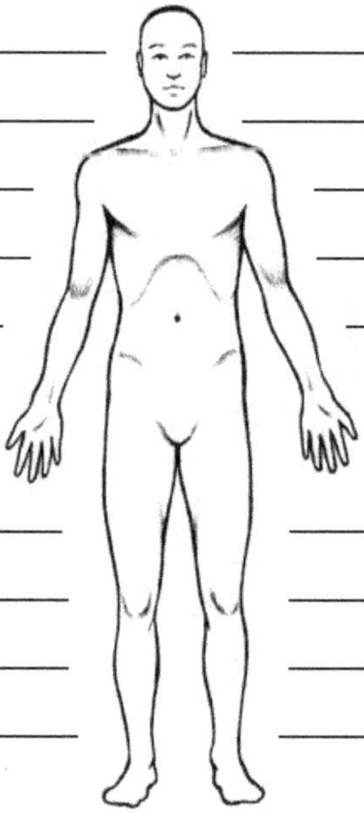

TRUST YOUR HEART ♥ TRUST YOUR HEART

TRUST YOUR HEART ♥ TRUST YOUR HEART ♥

TRUST YOUR HEART ♥ TRUST YOUR HEART ♥ TRUST YOUR HEART

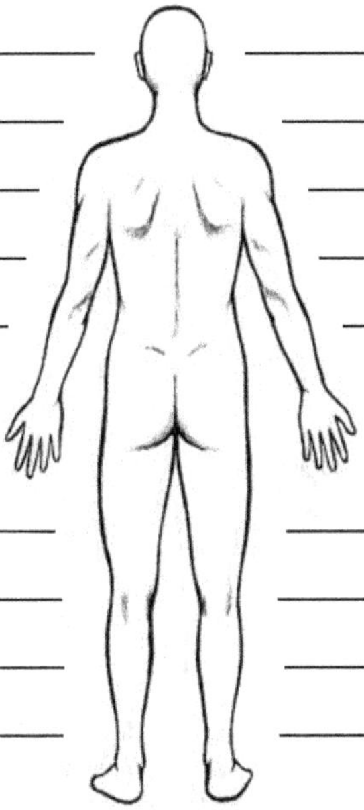

TRUST YOUR HEART ♥ TRUST YOUR HEART ♥

SHOULDERS: RESPONSIBILITY ♥ SHOULDERS: RESPONSIBILITY

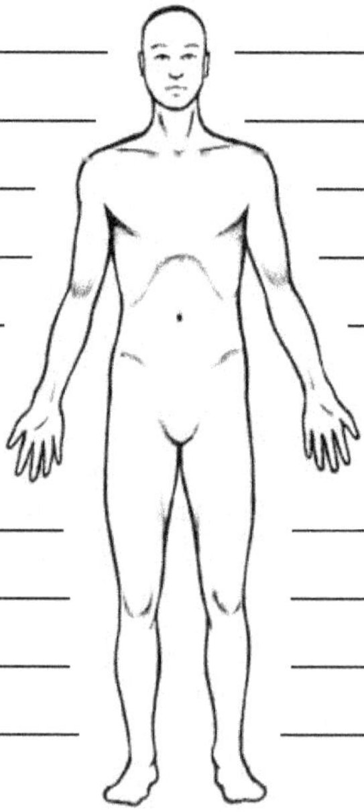

SHOULDERS: RESPONSIBILITY ♥ SHOULDERS: RESPONSIBILITY

SHOULDERS: RESPONSIBILITY ♥ SHOULDERS: RESPONSIBILITY

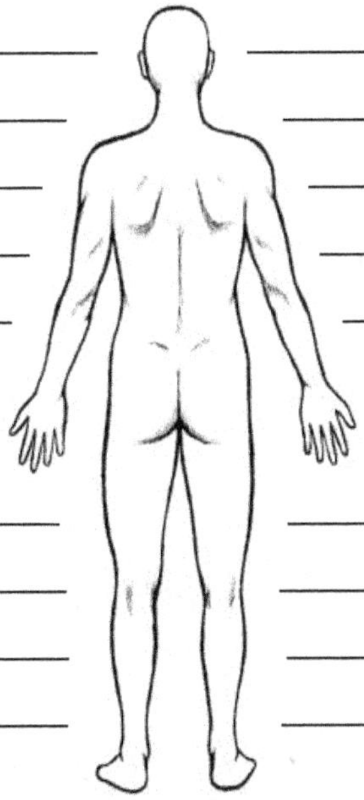

RESPONSE-ABILITY ♥ RESPONSE-ABILITY

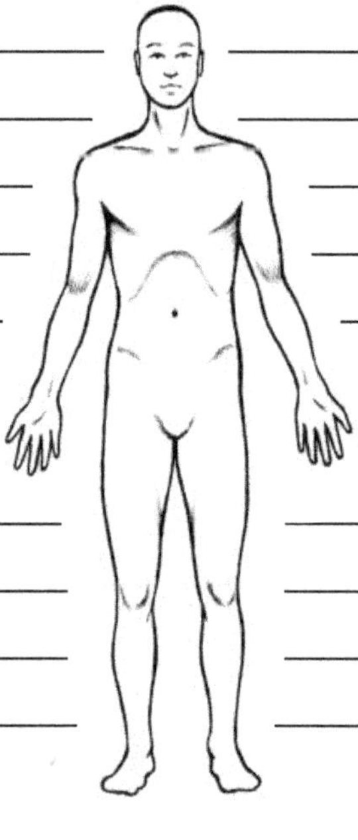

RESPONSE-ABILITY ♥ RESPONSE-ABILITY ♥

RESPONSE-ABILITY ♥ RESPONSE-ABILITY

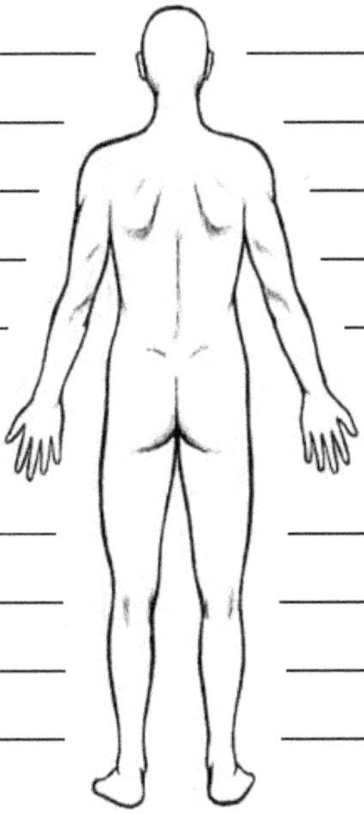

RESPONSE-ABILITY ♥ RESPONSE-ABILITY ♥

ARMS: EMBRACE ♥ ARMS: EMBRACE ♥ ARMS: EMBRACE

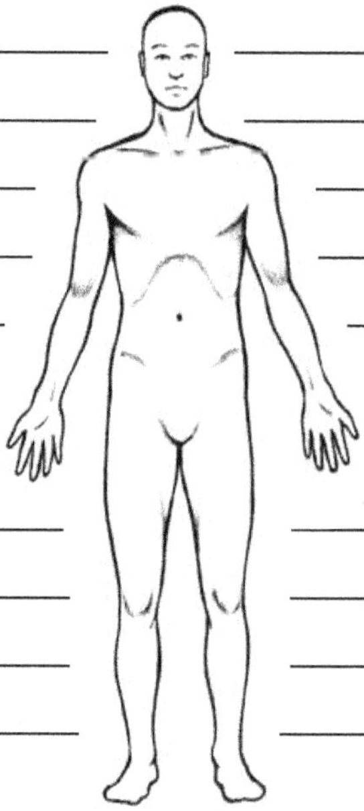

ARMS: EMBRACE ♥ ARMS: EMBRACE

ARMS: EMBRACE ♥ ARMS: EMBRACE ♥ ARMS: EMBRACE

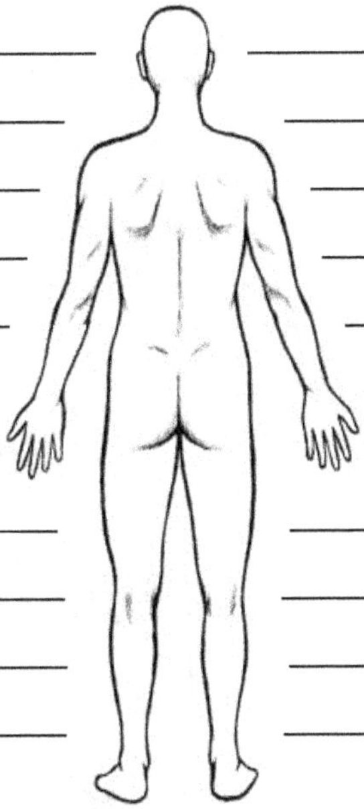

EMBRACE ALL THAT YOU FEEL ♥ EMBRACE ALL THAT YOU FEEL

EMBRACE ALL THAT YOU FEEL ♥ EMBRACE ALL THAT YOU FEEL

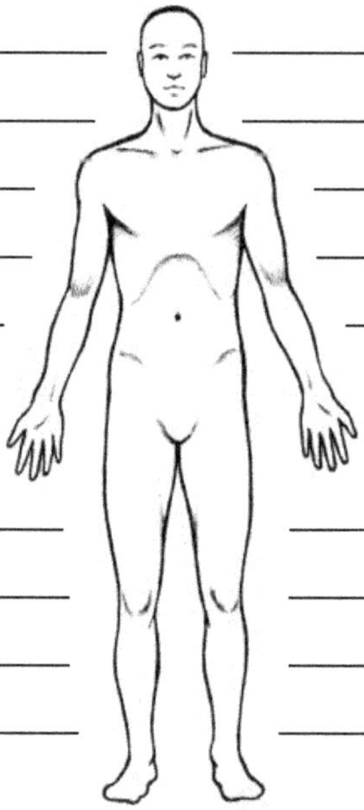

EMBRACE ALL THAT YOU FEEL ♥ EMBRACE ALL THAT YOU FEEL

EMBRACE ALL THAT YOU FEEL ♥ EMBRACE ALL THAT YOU FEEL ♥

EMBRACE ALL THAT YOU FEEL ♥ EMBRACE ALL THAT YOU FEEL

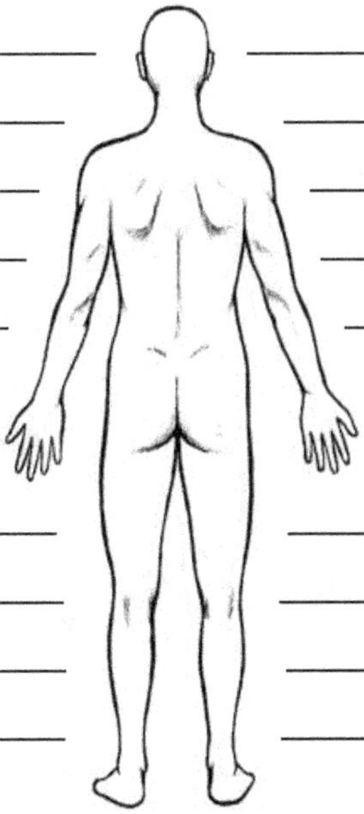

EMBRACE ALL THAT YOU FEEL ♥ EMBRACE ALL THAT YOU FEEL ♥

HANDS: GIVE & RECEIVE ♥ HANDS: GIVE & RECEIVE ♥ HANDS: GIVE & RECEIVE

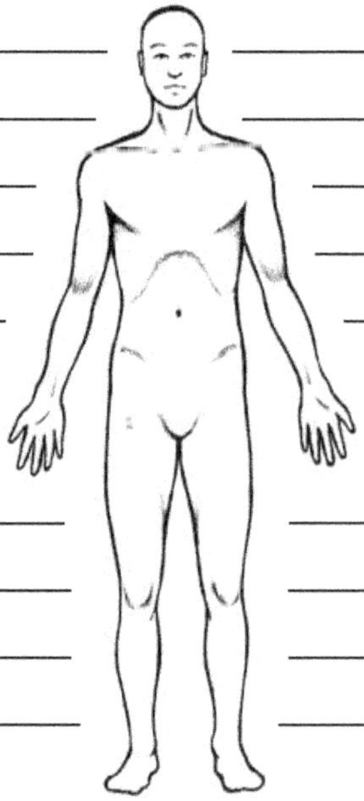

HANDS: GIVE & RECEIVE ❤ HANDS: GIVE & RECEIVE ❤ HANDS: GIVE & RECEIVE

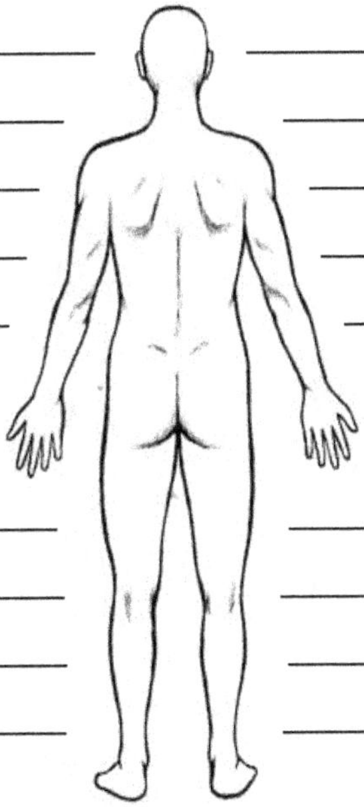

HANDS: GIVE & RECEIVE ❤ HANDS: GIVE & RECEIVE ❤

GIVING IS RECEIVING ♥ RECEIVING IS GIVING

RECEIVING IS GIVING ♥ GIVING IS RECEIVING

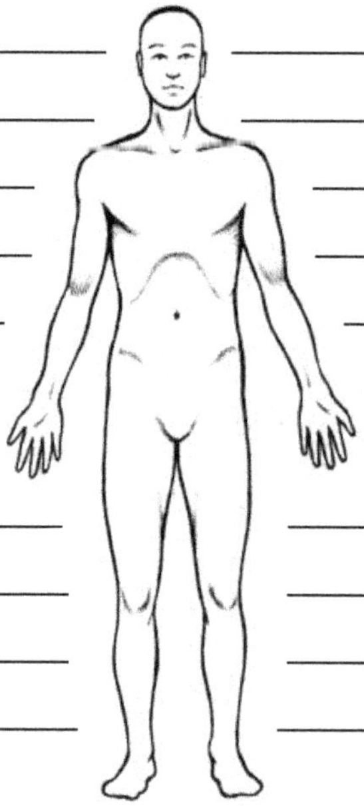

GIVING IS RECEIVING ♥ RECEIVING IS GIVING

GIVING IS RECEIVING ♥ RECEIVING IS GIVING ♥

GIVING IS RECEIVING ♥ RECEIVING IS GIVING

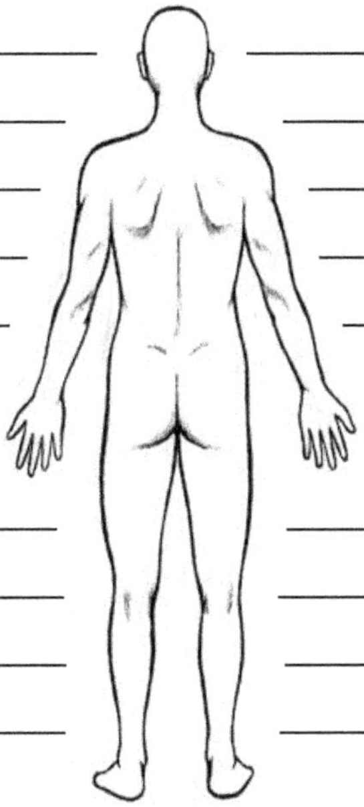

GIVING IS RECEIVING ♥ RECEIVING IS GIVING ♥

NECK: PATH OF COMMUNICATION BETWEEN HEAD & HEART

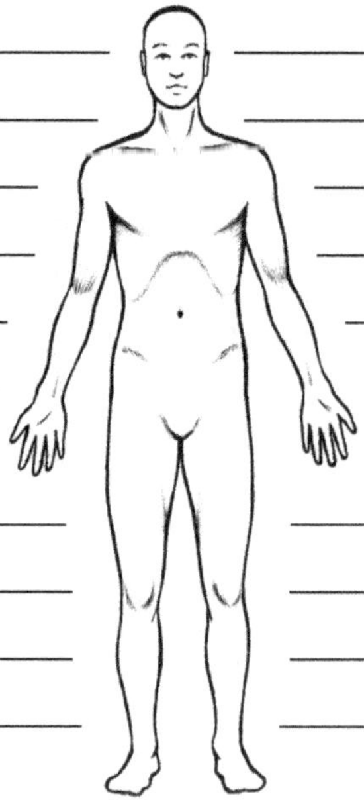

NECK: PATH OF COMMUNICATION BETWEEN HEAD & HEART

NECK: PATH OF COMMUNICATION BETWEEN HEAD & HEART

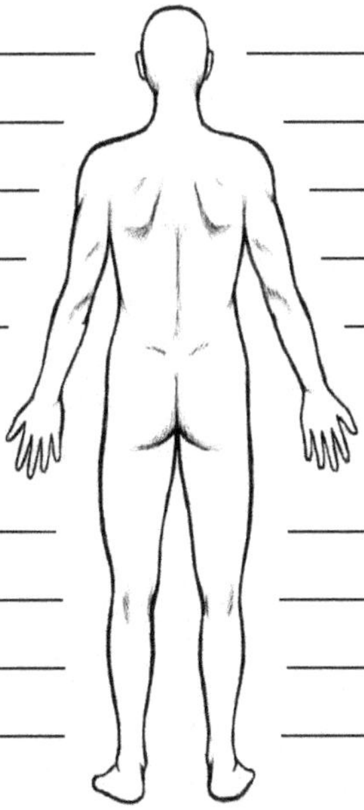

NECK: PATH OF COMMUNICATION BETWEEN HEAD & HEART

SPEAK THE WISDOM OF YOUR HEART ♥ SPEAK THE WISDOM OF YOUR HEART

SPEAK THE WISDOM OF YOUR HEART ♥ SPEAK THE WISDOM OF YOUR HEART

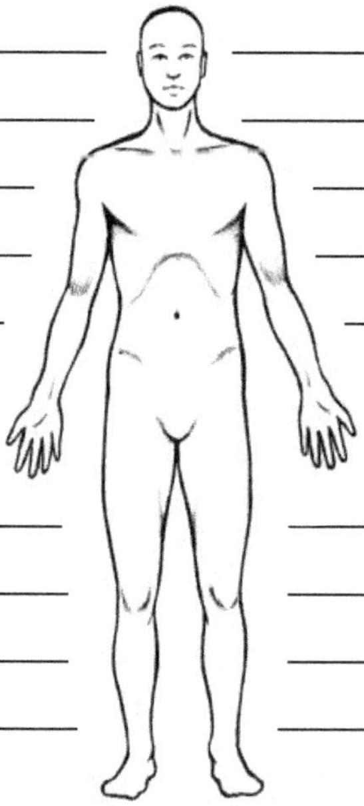

SPEAK THE WISDOM OF YOUR HEART ♥ SPEAK THE WISDOM OF YOUR HEART

SPEAK THE WISDOM OF YOUR HEART ♥ SPEAK THE WISDOM OF YOUR HEART ♥

SPEAK THE WISDOM OF YOUR HEART ♥ SPEAK THE WISDOM OF YOUR HEART

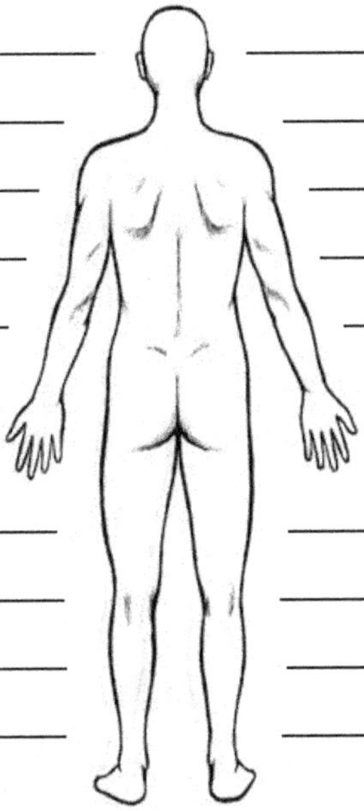

SPEAK THE WISDOM OF YOUR HEART ♥ SPEAK THE WISDOM OF YOUR HEART ♥

HEAD: WHERE YOU HOLD YOUR THOUGHTS ♥ HEAD: WHERE YOU HOLD YOUR THOUGHTS

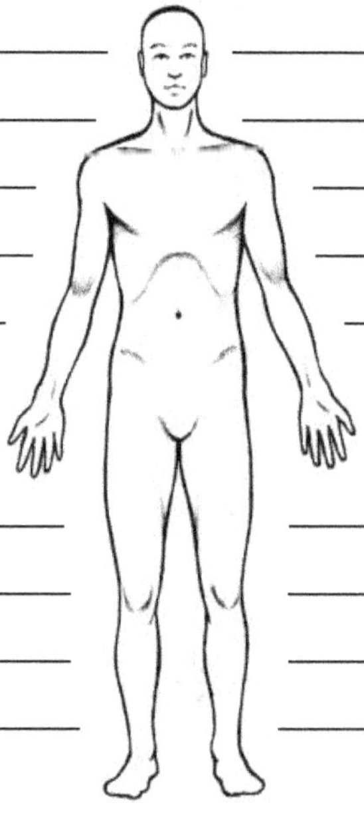

HEAD: WHERE YOU HOLD YOUR THOUGHTS ♥ HEAD: WHERE YOU HOLD YOUR THOUGHTS

HEAD: WHERE YOU HOLD YOUR THOUGHTS ♥ HEAD: WHERE YOU HOLD YOUR THOUGHTS

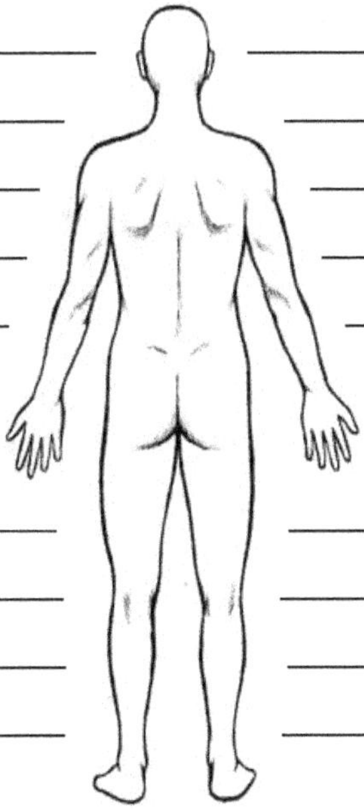

HEAD: WHERE YOU HOLD YOUR THOUGHTS ♥ HEAD: WHERE YOU HOLD YOUR THOUGHTS ♥

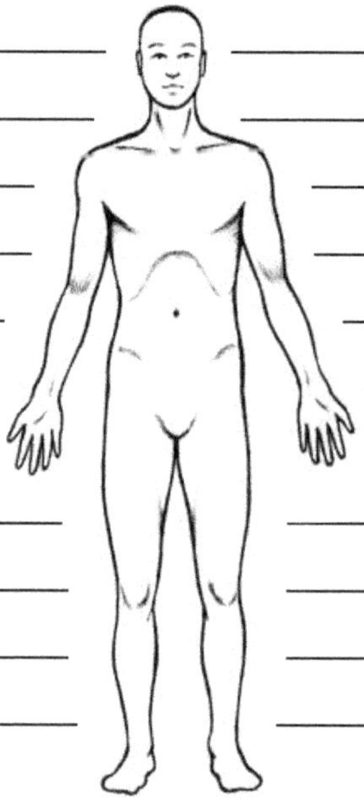

KNOW YOUR WISDOM ♥ KNOW YOUR WISDOM ♥ KNOW YOUR WISDOM

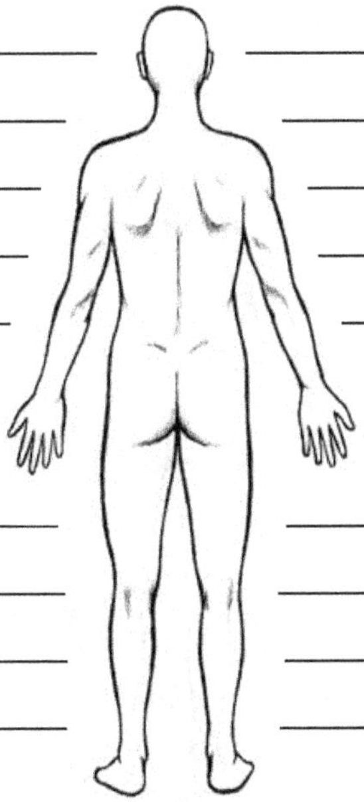

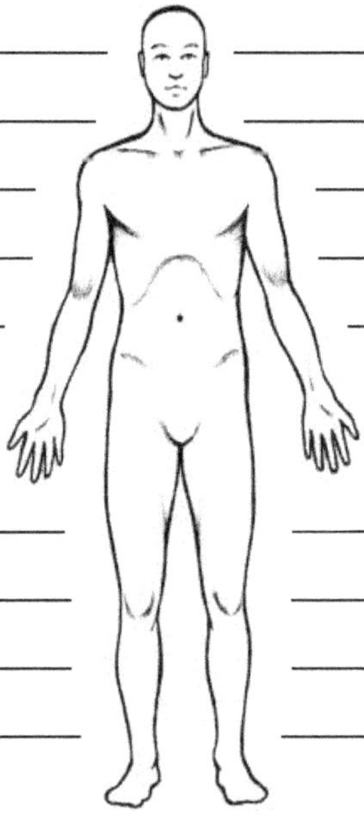

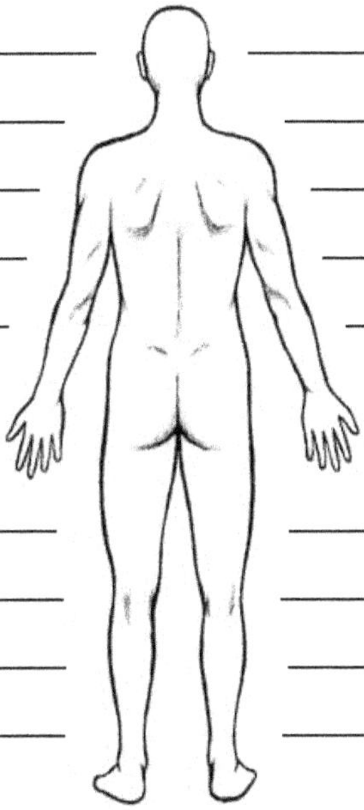

FACE THE WORLD FROM WITHIN ♥ FACE THE WORLD FROM WITHIN

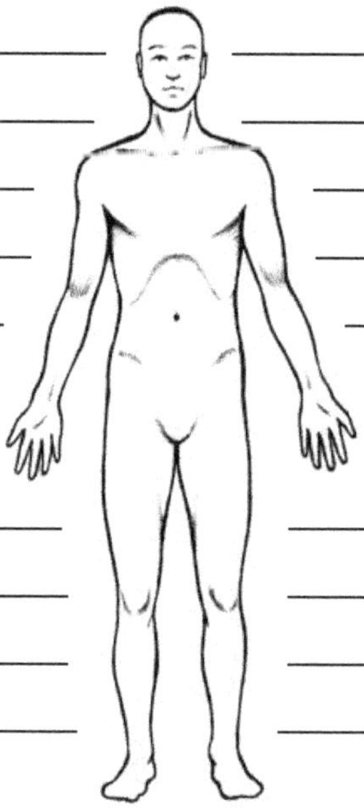

FACE THE WORLD FROM WITHIN ♥ FACE THE WORLD FROM WITHIN

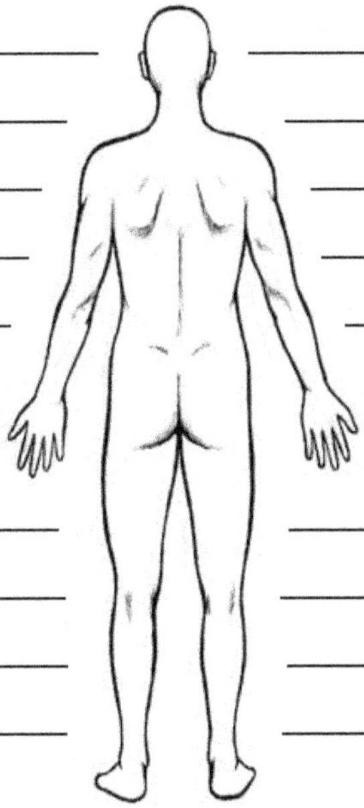

ENJOY THE JOURNEY ♥ ENJOY THE JOURNEY

ENJOY THE JOURNEY ♥ ENJOY THE JOURNEY ♥ ENJOY THE JOURNEY

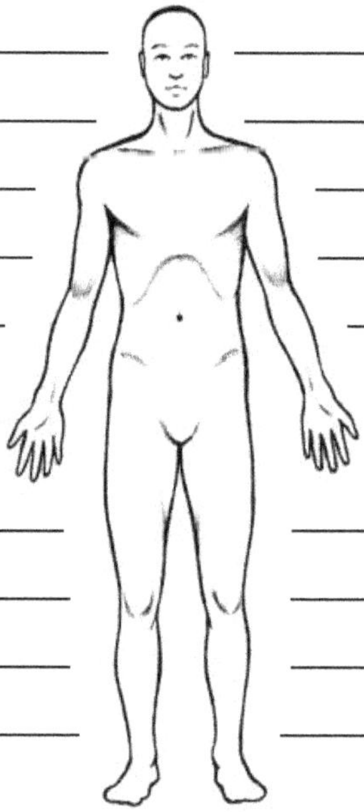

ENJOY THE JOURNEY ♥ ENJOY THE JOURNEY

ENJOY THE JOURNEY ♥ ENJOY THE JOURNEY ♥ ENJOY THE JOURNEY

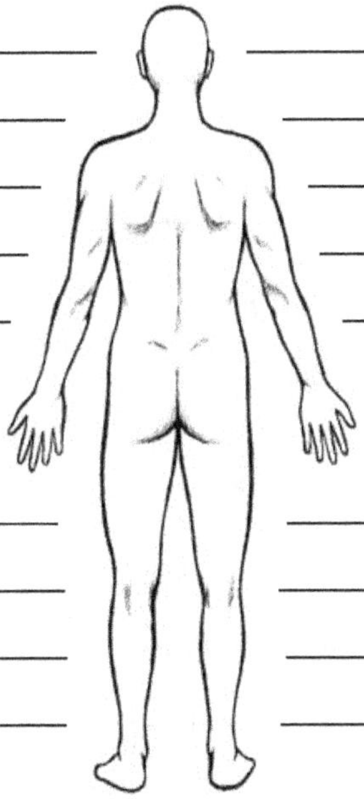

ASK YOURSELF QUESTIONS ♥ ASK YOURSELF QUESTIONS

ASK YOURSELF QUESTIONS ♥ ASK YOURSELF QUESTIONS

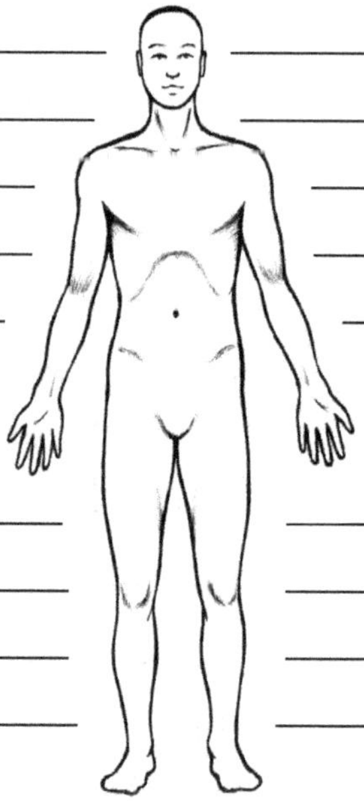

ASK YOURSELF QUESTIONS ♥ ASK YOURSELF QUESTIONS

ASK YOURSELF QUESTIONS ♥ ASK YOURSELF QUESTIONS

ASK YOURSELF QUESTIONS ♥ ASK YOURSELF QUESTIONS

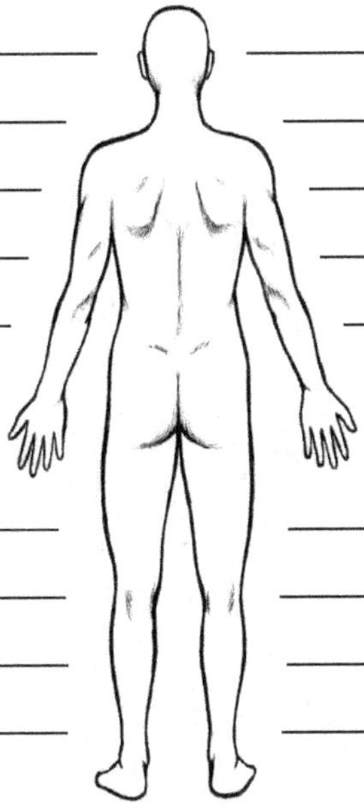

ASK YOURSELF QUESTIONS ♥ ASK YOURSELF QUESTIONS

SEEK THE ANSWER WITHIN ♥ SEEK THE ANSWER WITHIN

SEEK THE ANSWER WITHIN ♥ SEEK THE ANSWER WITHIN

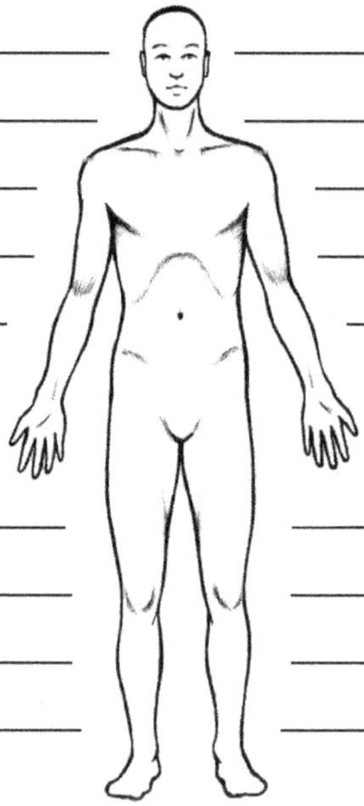

SEEK THE ANSWER WITHIN ♥ SEEK THE ANSWER WITHIN

SEEK THE ANSWER WITHIN ♥ SEEK THE ANSWER WITHIN ♥

SEEK THE ANSWER WITHIN ♥ SEEK THE ANSWER WITHIN

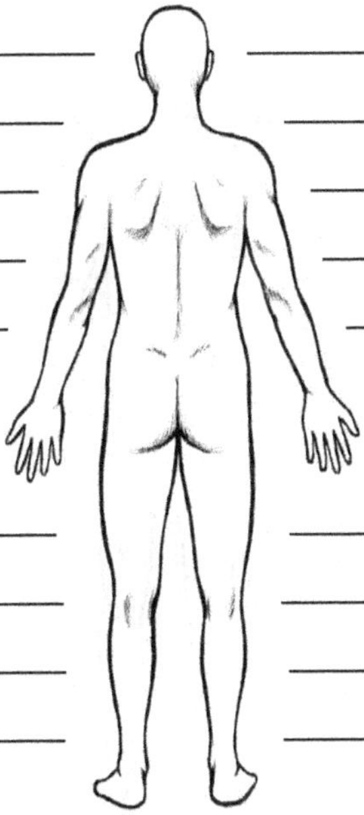

SEEK THE ANSWER WITHIN ♥ SEEK THE ANSWER WITHIN ♥

FEET: FOUNDATION ♥ FEET: FOUNDATION ♥ FEET: FOUNDATION

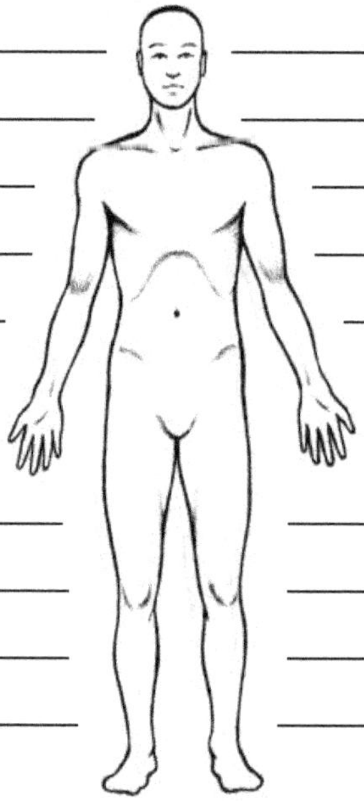

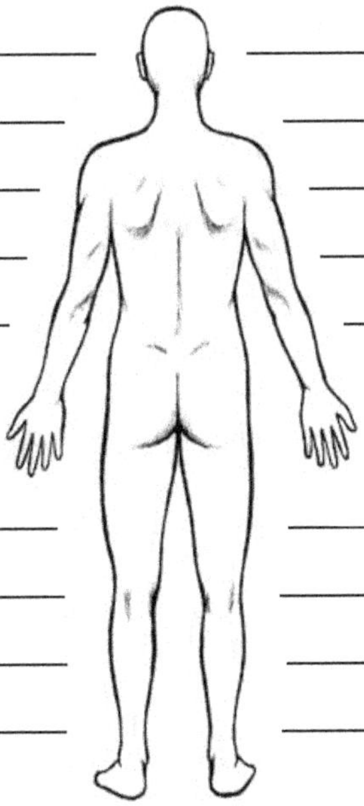

BE CURIOUS ♥ BE CURIOUS

BE CURIOUS ♥ BE CURIOUS ♥ BE CURIOUS

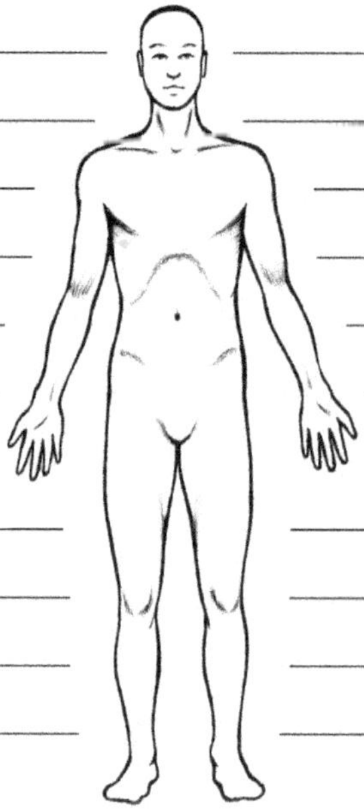

BE CURIOUS ♥ BE CURIOUS

B E C U R I O U S ❤ B E C U R I O U S ❤ B E C U R I O U S

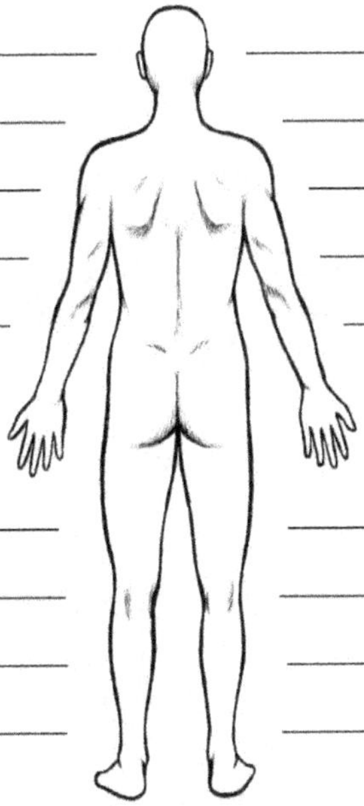

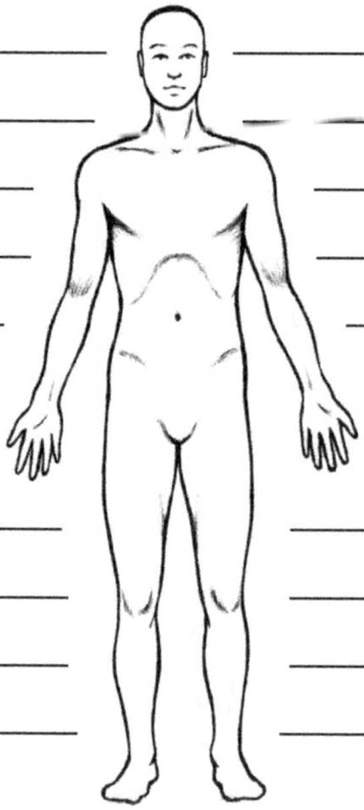

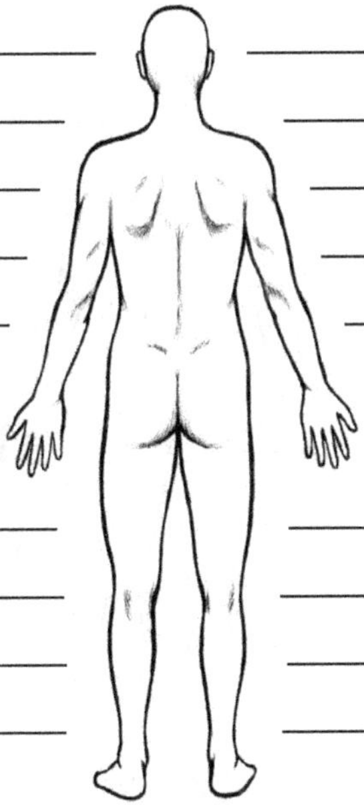

JOINTS: ARTICULATE MOVEMENT
JOINTS: ARTICULATE MOVEMENT

MOVE INTO YOURSELF ♥ MOVE INTO YOURSELF ♥ MOVE INTO YOURSELF

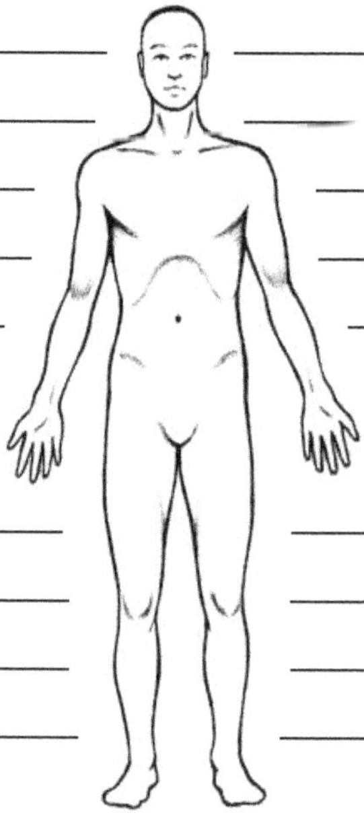

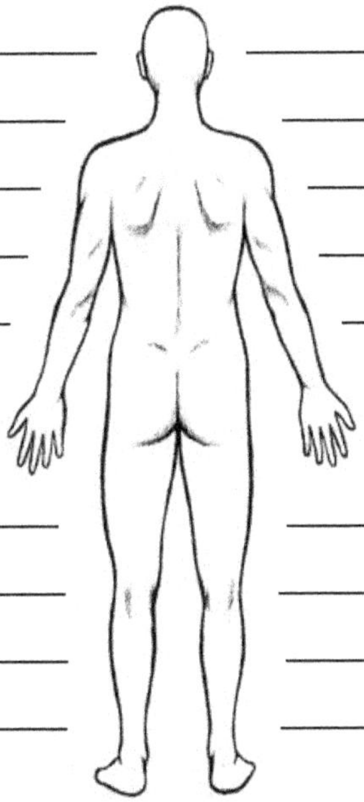

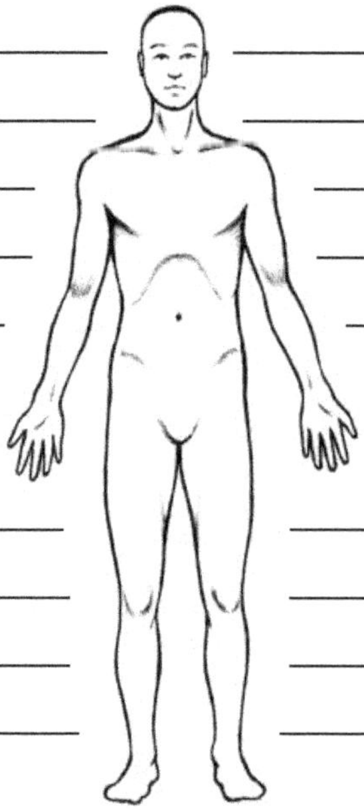

LEGS: HOW YOU STAND & MOVE ♥ LEGS: HOW YOU STAND & MOVE

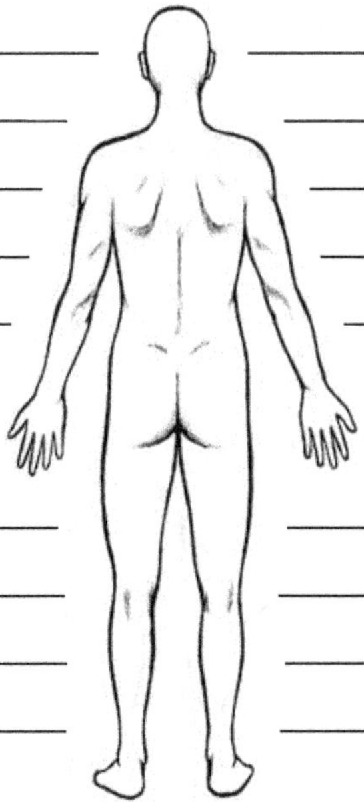

FOLLOW THE FEELINGS ♥ FOLLOW THE FEELINGS

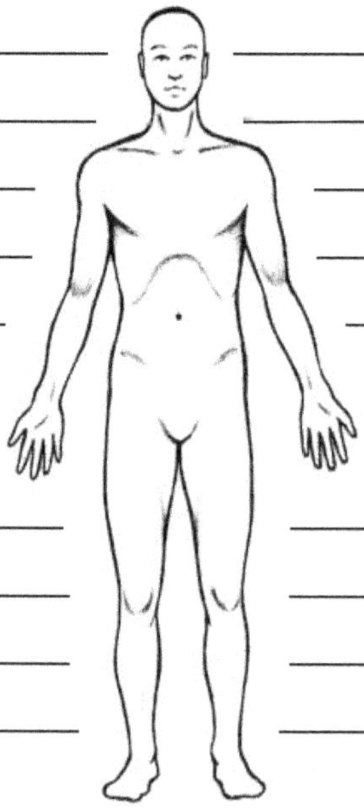

FOLLOW THE FEELINGS ♥ FOLLOW THE FEELINGS

FOLLOW THE FEELINGS ♥ FOLLOW THE FEELINGS ♥

FOLLOW THE FEELINGS ♥ FOLLOW THE FEELINGS

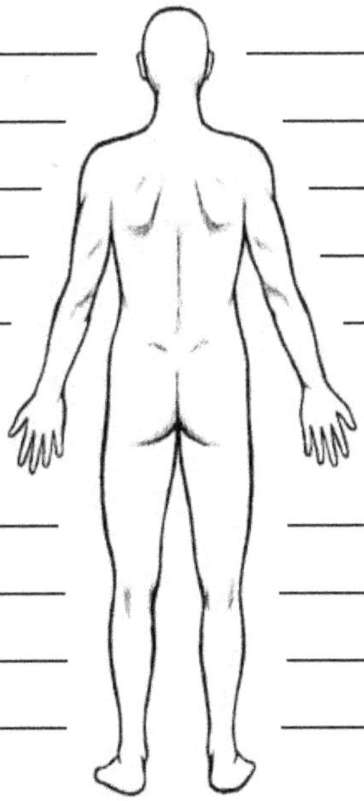

FOLLOW THE FEELINGS ♥ FOLLOW THE FEELINGS ♥

PELVIS: CREATIVE LIFE FORCE ♥ PELVIS: CREATIVE LIFE FORCE

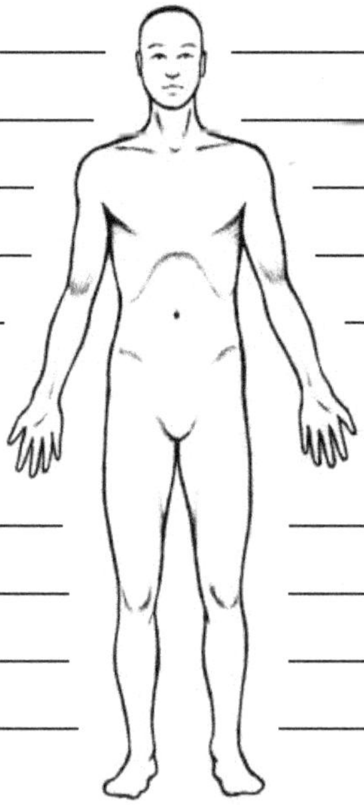

PELVIS: CREATIVE LIFE FORCE ♥ PELVIS: CREATIVE LIFE FORCE

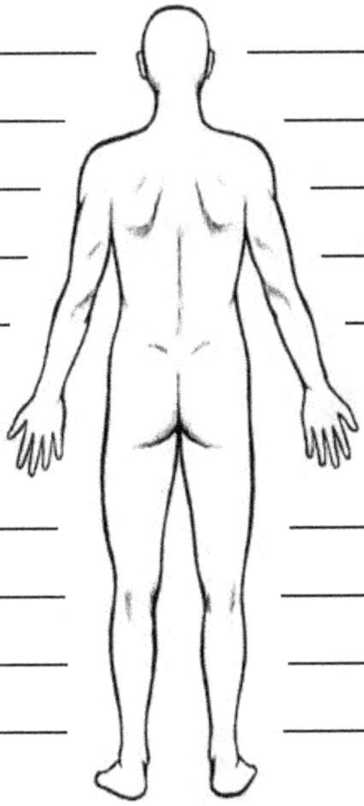

EXPLORE THE EXPERIENCE ♥ EXPLORE THE EXPERIENCE

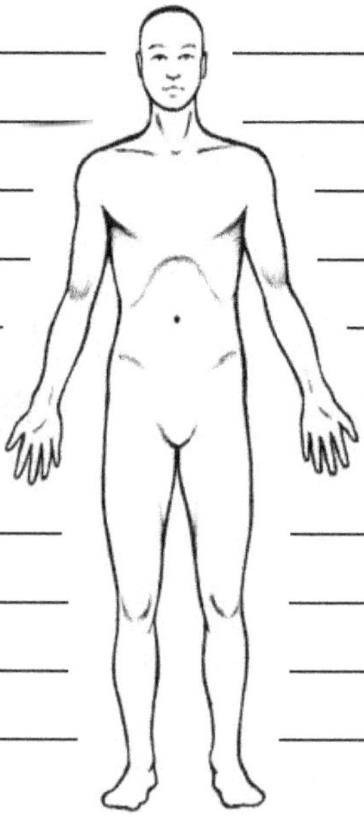

EXPLORE THE EXPERIENCE ♥ EXPLORE THE EXPERIENCE

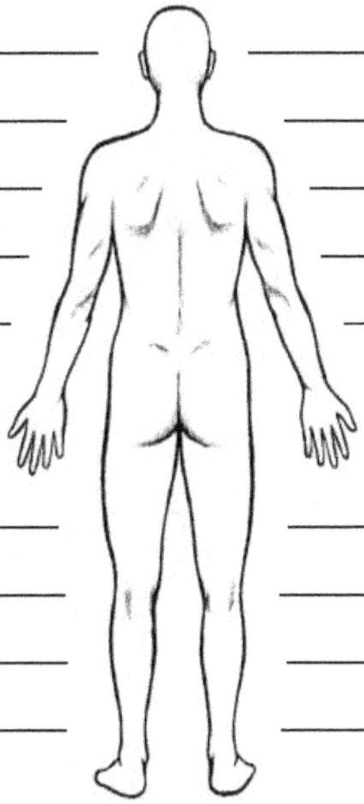

BELLY: EMOTIONAL CENTER ♥ BELLY: EMOTIONAL CENTER ♥ BELLY: EMOTIONAL CENTER

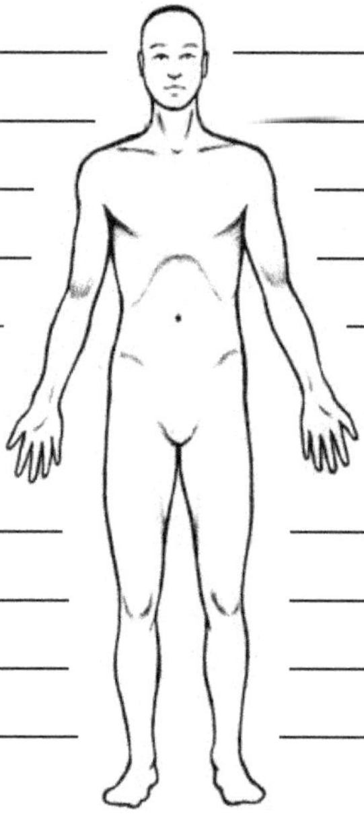

BELLY: EMOTIONAL CENTER ♥ BELLY: EMOTIONAL CENTER

BELLY: EMOTIONAL CENTER ♥ BELLY: EMOTIONAL CENTER ♥ BELLY: EMOTIONAL CENTER

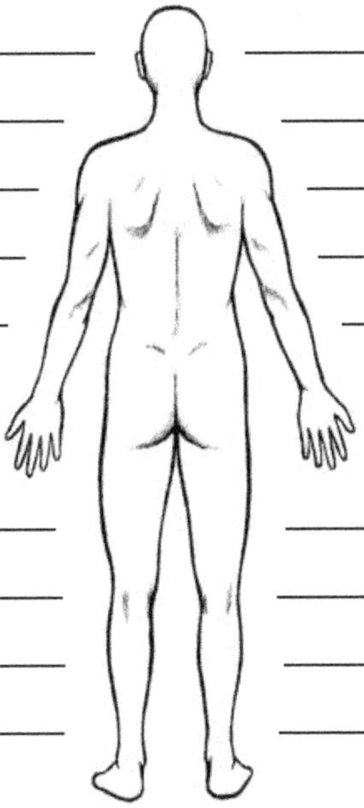

ANSWER TO YOUR FEELINGS ♥ ANSWER TO YOUR FEELINGS

ANSWER TO YOUR FEELINGS ♥ ANSWER TO YOUR FEELINGS

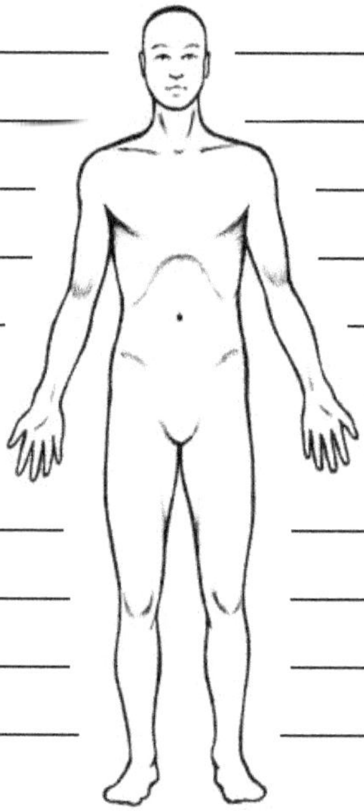

ANSWER TO YOUR FEELINGS ♥ ANSWER TO YOUR FEELINGS

ANSWER TO YOUR FEELINGS ♥ ANSWER TO YOUR FEELINGS

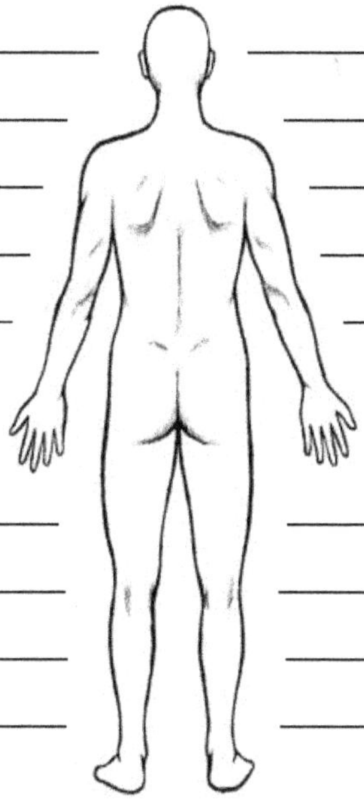

ANSWER TO YOUR FEELINGS ♥ ANSWER TO YOUR FEELINGS ♥

CHEST: HEART CENTER ❤ CHEST: HEART CENTER ❤ CHEST: HEART CENTER

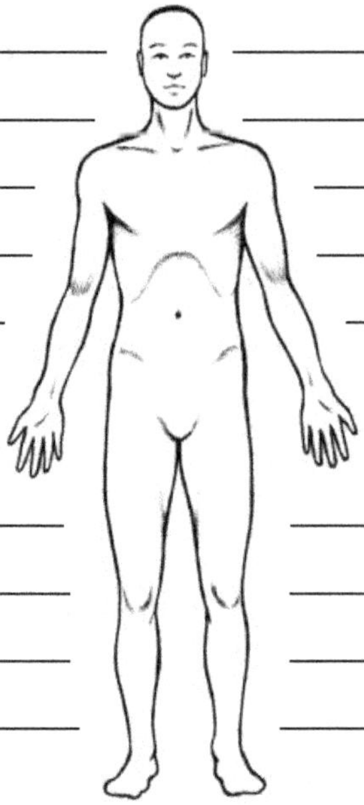

CHEST: HEART CENTER ♥ CHEST: HEART CENTER ♥ CHEST: HEART CENTER

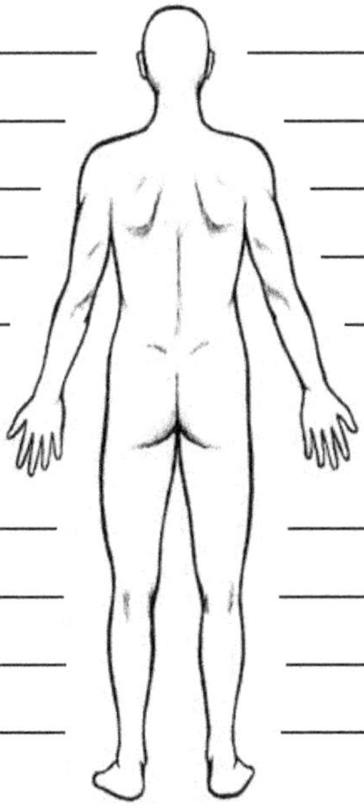

CHEST: HEART CENTER ♥ CHEST: HEART CENTER ♥

LEAD WITH YOUR HEART ♥ LEAD WITH YOUR HEART

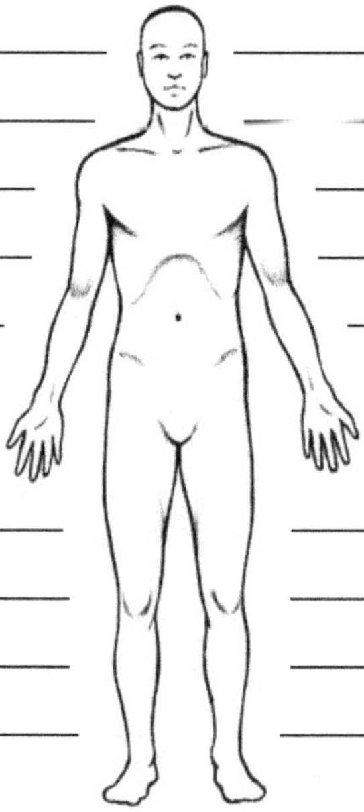

LEAD WITH YOUR HEART ♥ LEAD WITH YOUR HEART

LEAD WITH YOUR HEART ♥ LEAD WITH YOUR HEART ♥

LEAD WITH YOUR HEART ♥ LEAD WITH YOUR HEART

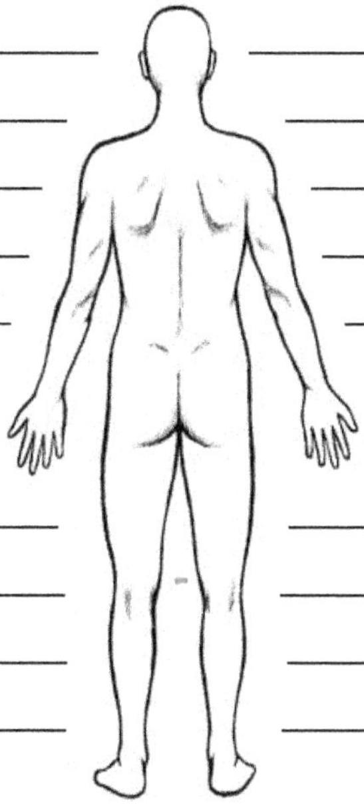

LEAD WITH YOUR HEART ♥ LEAD WITH YOUR HEART ♥

RIBS: HEART SUPPORT ♥ RIBS: HEART SUPPORT ♥ RIBS: HEART SUPPORT

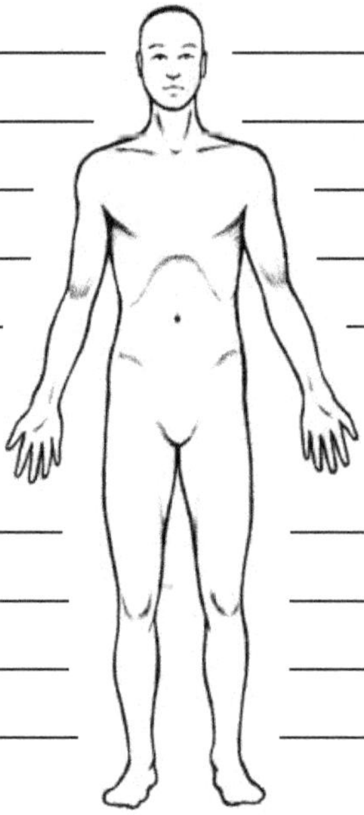

RIBS: HEART SUPPORT ♥ RIBS: HEART SUPPORT

RIBS: HEART SUPPORT ❤ RIBS: HEART SUPPORT ❤ RIBS: HEART SUPPORT

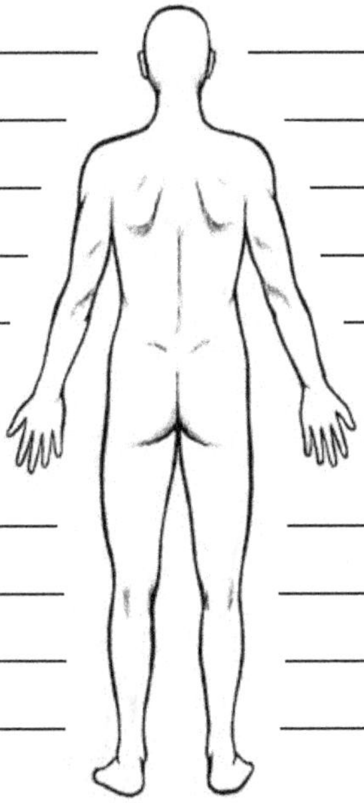

RIBS: HEART SUPPORT ❤ RIBS: HEART SUPPORT ❤

TRUST YOUR HEART ♥ TRUST YOUR HEART

TRUST YOUR HEART ♥ TRUST YOUR HEART ♥ TRUST YOUR HEART

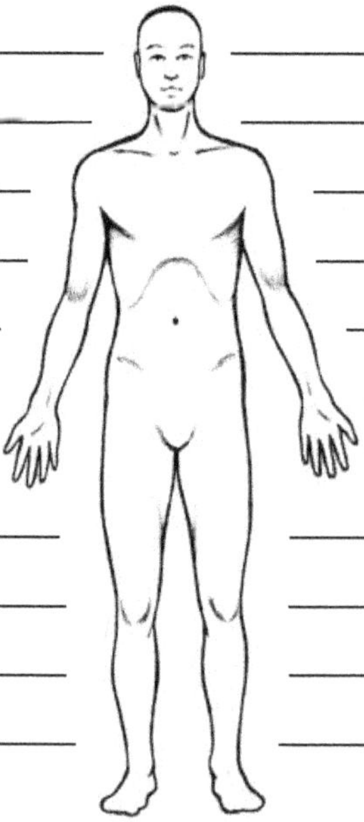

TRUST YOUR HEART ♥ TRUST YOUR HEART

TRUST YOUR HEART ♥ TRUST YOUR HEART ♥

TRUST YOUR HEART ♥ TRUST YOUR HEART ♥ TRUST YOUR HEART

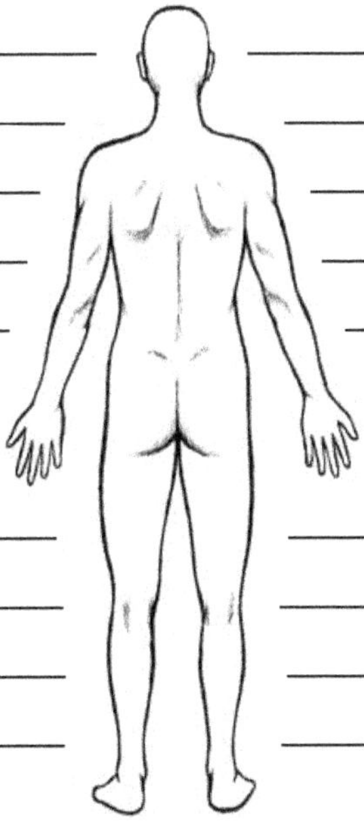

TRUST YOUR HEART ♥ TRUST YOUR HEART ♥

SHOULDERS: RESPONSIBILITY ♥ SHOULDERS: RESPONSIBILITY

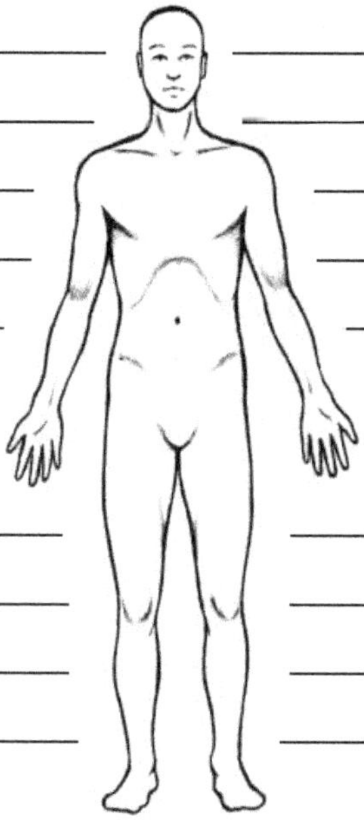

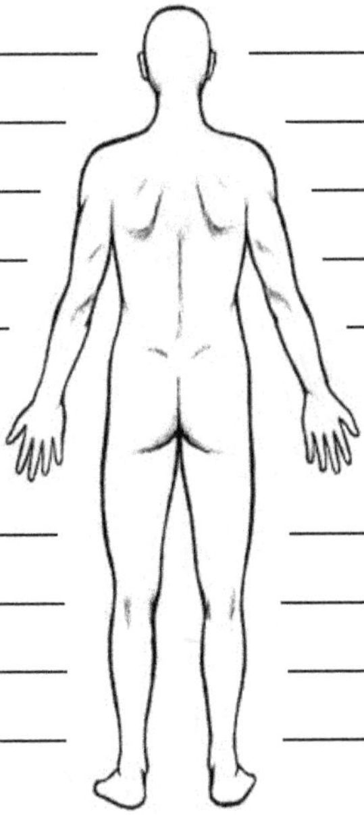

SHOULDERS: RESPONSIBILITY ♥ SHOULDERS: RESPONSIBILITY

♥ RESPONSE-ABILITY ♥ RESPONSE-ABILITY

RESPONSE-ABILITY ♥ RESPONSE-ABILITY

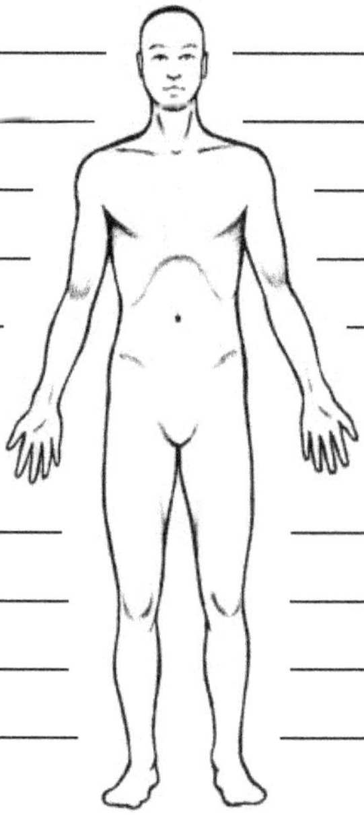

♥ RESPONSE-ABILITY ♥ RESPONSE-ABILITY

RESPONSE-ABILITY ♥ RESPONSE-ABILITY ♥

RESPONSE-ABILITY ♥ RESPONSE-ABILITY

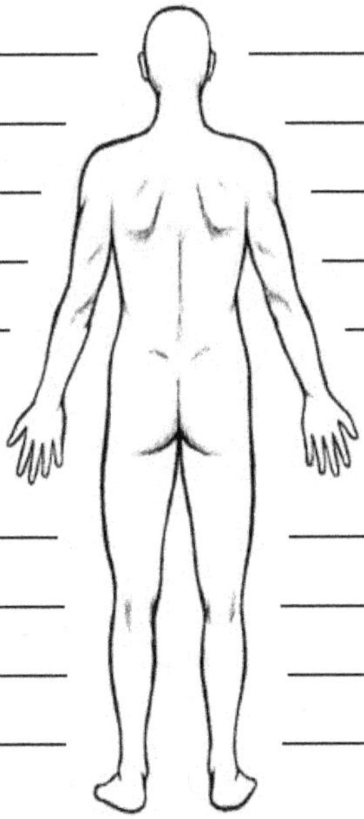

RESPONSE-ABILITY ♥ RESPONSE-ABILITY ♥

ARMS: EMBRACE

ARMS: EMBRACE
ARMS: EMBRACE
ARMS: EMBRACE
ARMS: EMBRACE

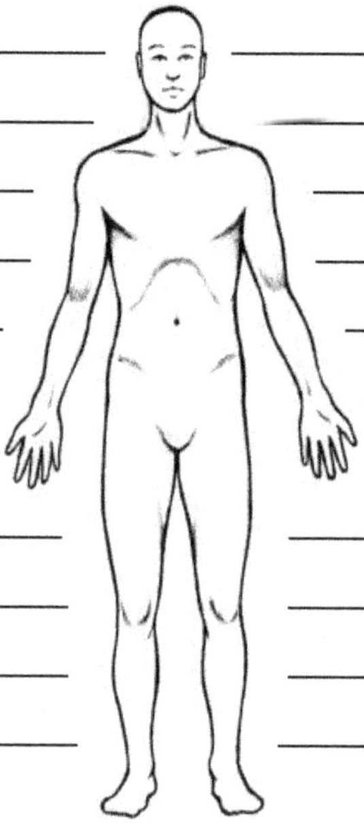

ARMS: EMBRACE
ARMS: EMBRACE
ARMS: EMBRACE
ARMS: EMBRACE

ARMS: EMBRACE ♥ ARMS: EMBRACE ♥ ARMS: EMBRACE

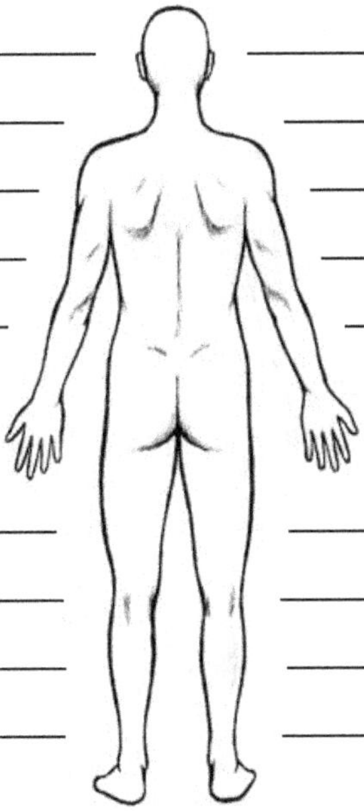

EMBRACE ALL THAT YOU FEEL ♥ EMBRACE ALL THAT YOU FEEL

EMBRACE ALL THAT YOU FEEL ♥ EMBRACE ALL THAT YOU FEEL

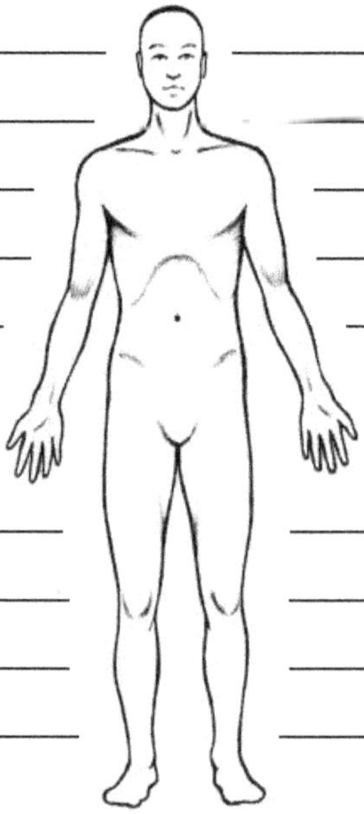

EMBRACE ALL THAT YOU FEEL ♥ EMBRACE ALL THAT YOU FEEL

EMBRACE ALL THAT YOU FEEL ♥ EMBRACE ALL THAT YOU FEEL

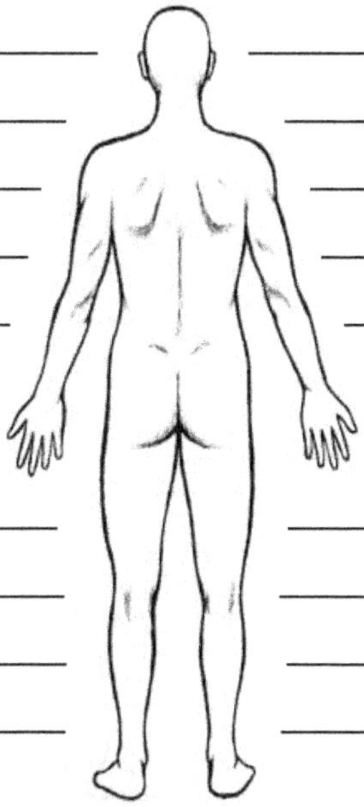

HANDS: GIVE & RECEIVE
HANDS: GIVE & RECEIVE
HANDS: GIVE & RECEIVE
HANDS: GIVE & RECEIVE

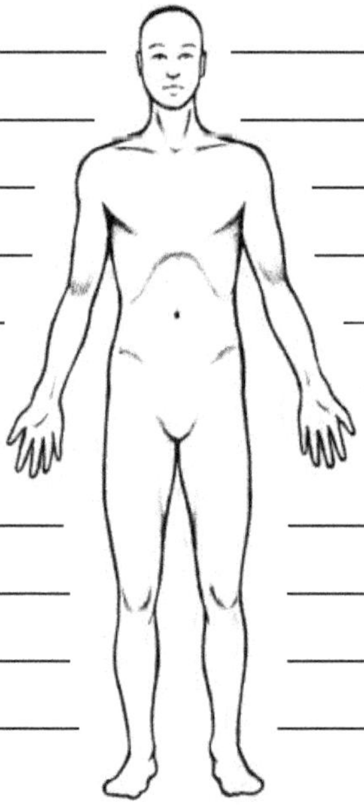

HANDS: GIVE & RECEIVE
HANDS: GIVE & RECEIVE

HANDS: GIVE & RECEIVE ♥ HANDS: GIVE & RECEIVE ♥ HANDS: GIVE & RECEIVE

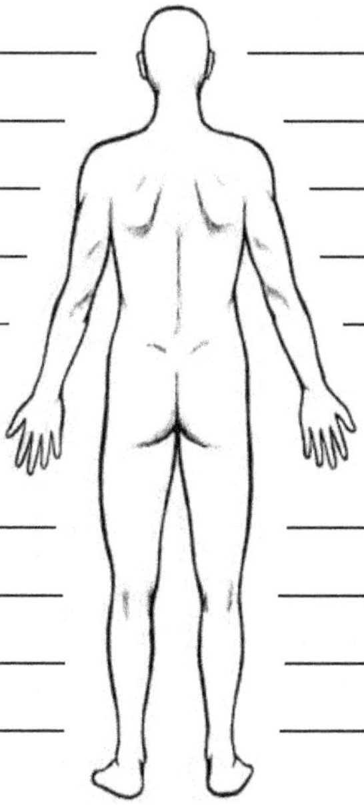

GIVING IS RECEIVING ♥ RECEIVING IS GIVING

RECEIVING IS GIVING

GIVING IS RECEIVING

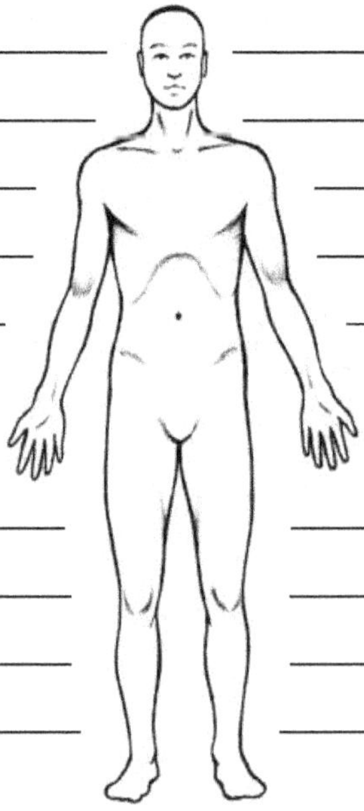

GIVING IS RECEIVING ♥ RECEIVING IS GIVING

GIVING IS RECEIVING ♥ RECEIVING IS GIVING ♥

GIVING IS RECEIVING ♥ RECEIVING IS GIVING

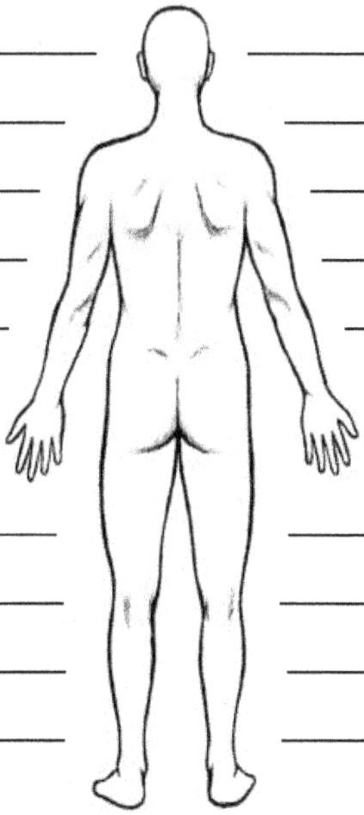

GIVING IS RECEIVING ♥ RECEIVING IS GIVING ♥

NECK: PATH OF COMMUNICATION BETWEEN HEAD & HEART

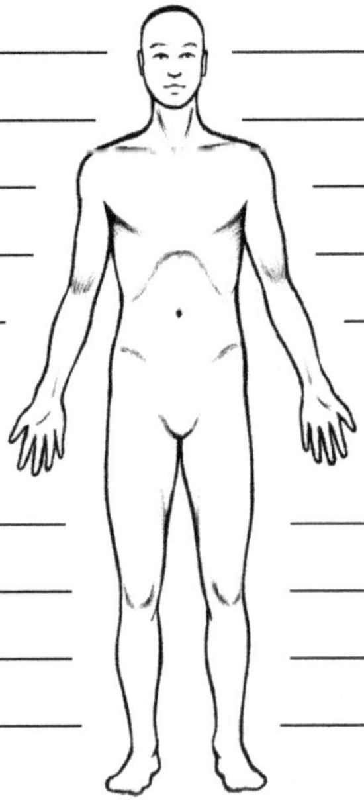

NECK: PATH OF COMMUNICATION BETWEEN HEAD & HEART

NECK: PATH OF COMMUNICATION BETWEEN HEAD & HEART

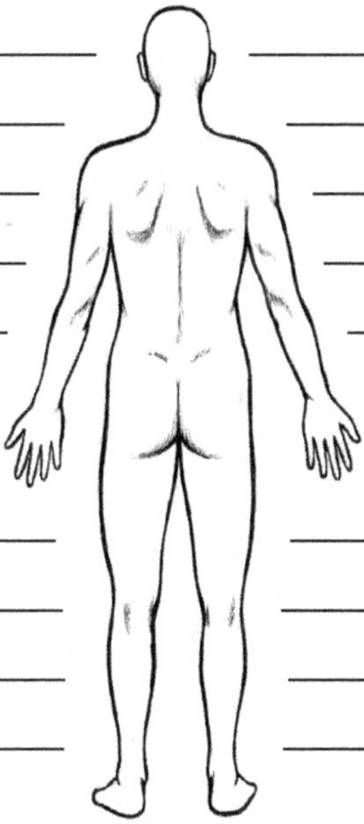

SPEAK THE WISDOM OF YOUR HEART ♥ SPEAK THE WISDOM OF YOUR HEART

SPEAK THE WISDOM OF YOUR HEART ♥ SPEAK THE WISDOM OF YOUR HEART

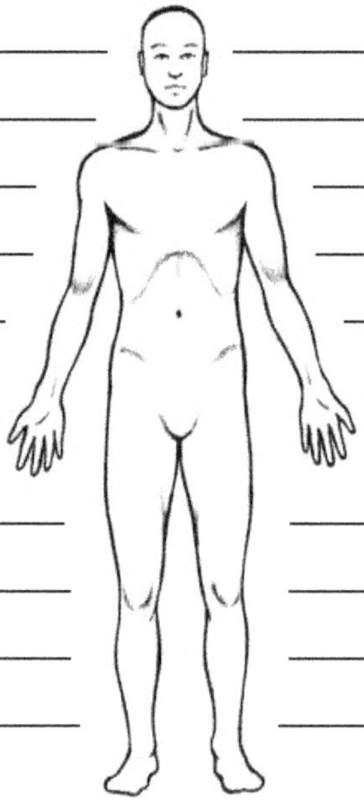

SPEAK THE WISDOM OF YOUR HEART ♥ SPEAK THE WISDOM OF YOUR HEART

SPEAK THE WISDOM OF YOUR HEART ♥ SPEAK THE WISDOM OF YOUR HEART

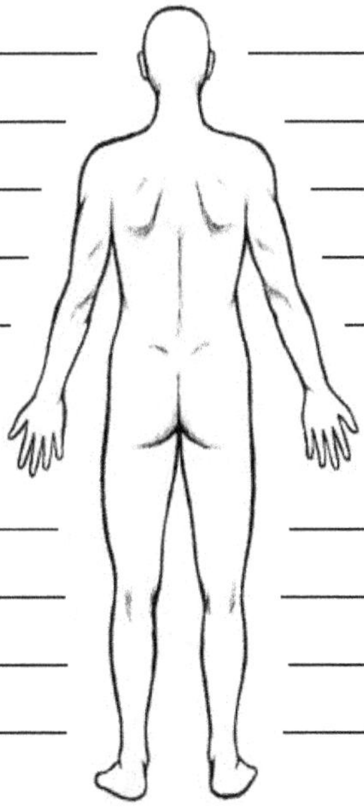

HEAD: WHERE YOU HOLD YOUR THOUGHTS ♥ HEAD: WHERE YOU HOLD YOUR THOUGHTS

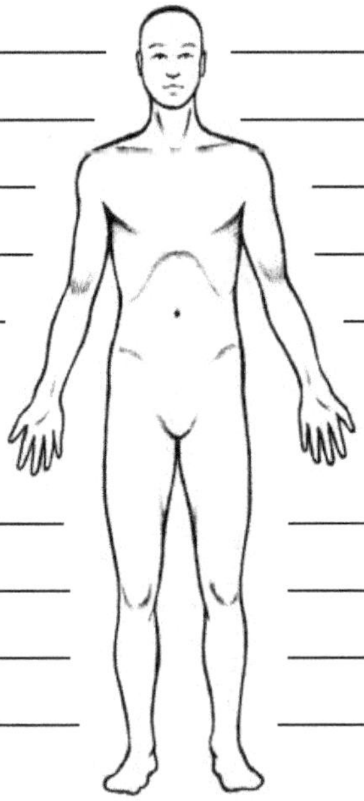

HEAD: WHERE YOU HOLD YOUR THOUGHTS ♥ HEAD: WHERE YOU HOLD YOUR THOUGHTS

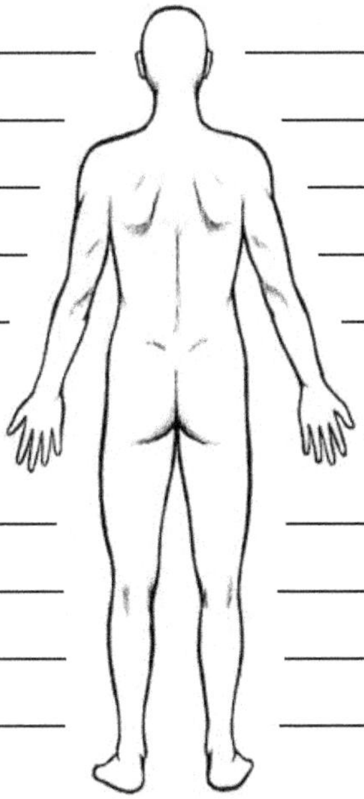

HEAD: WHERE YOU HOLD YOUR THOUGHTS ♥ HEAD: WHERE YOU HOLD YOUR THOUGHTS ♥

KNOW YOUR WISDOM ♥ KNOW YOUR WISDOM

KNOW YOUR WISDOM ♥ KNOW YOUR WISDOM ♥ KNOW YOUR WISDOM

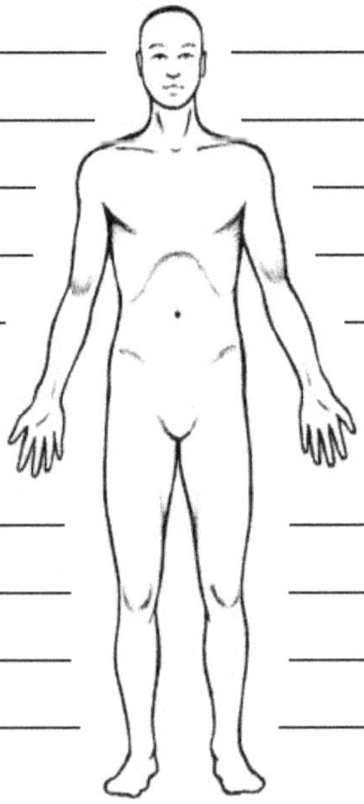

KNOW YOUR WISDOM ♥ KNOW YOUR WISDOM

KNOW YOUR WISDOM ♥ KNOW YOUR WISDOM ♥ KNOW YOUR WISDOM

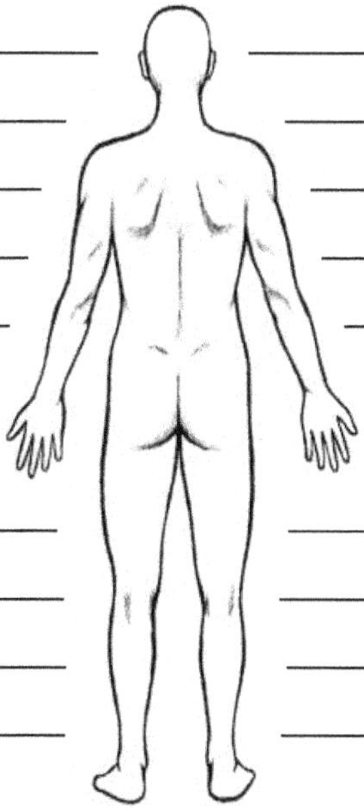

FACE: HOW YOU FACE THE WORLD ♥ FACE: HOW YOU FACE THE WORLD ♥ FACE: HOW YOU FACE THE WORLD

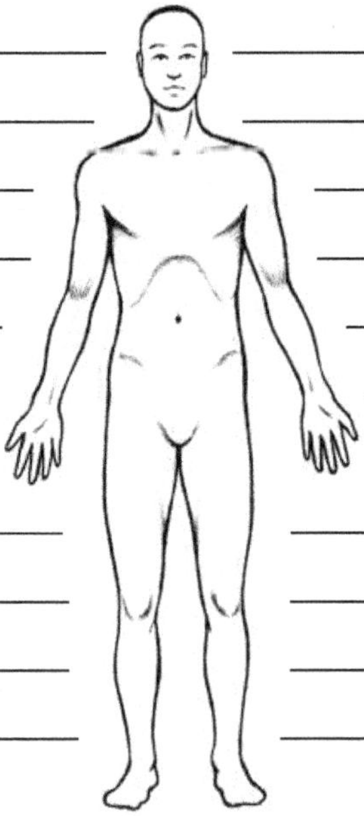

FACE: HOW YOU FACE THE WORLD ♥ FACE: HOW YOU FACE THE WORLD ♥ FACE: HOW YOU FACE THE WORLD

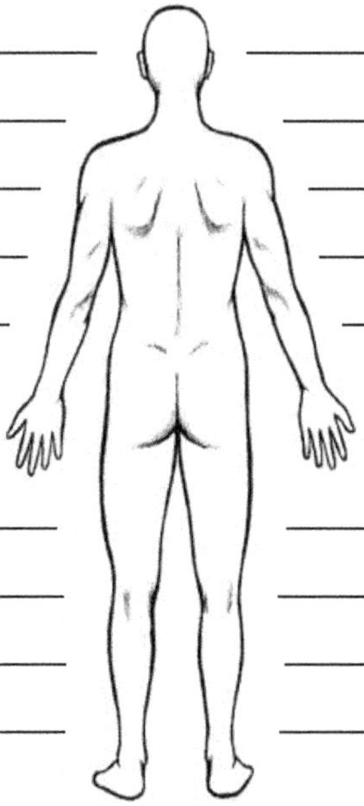

FACE THE WORLD FROM WITHIN ♥ FACE THE WORLD FROM WITHIN

FACE THE WORLD FROM WITHIN ♥ FACE THE WORLD FROM WITHIN

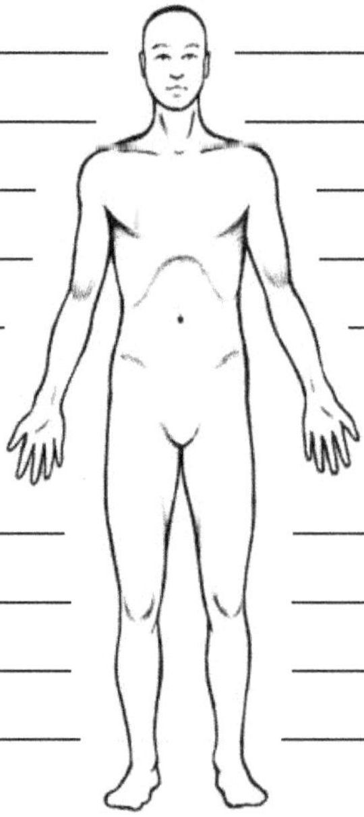

FACE THE WORLD FROM WITHIN ♥ FACE THE WORLD FROM WITHIN

FACE THE WORLD FROM WITHIN ♥ FACE THE WORLD FROM WITHIN

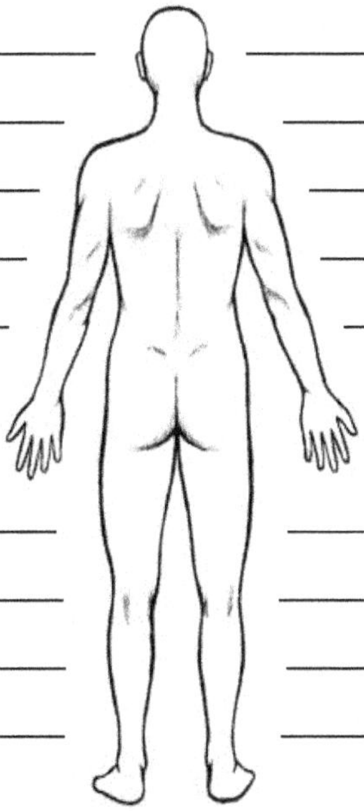

ENJOY THE JOURNEY ♥ ENJOY THE JOURNEY

ENJOY THE JOURNEY ♥ ENJOY THE JOURNEY ♥ ENJOY THE JOURNEY

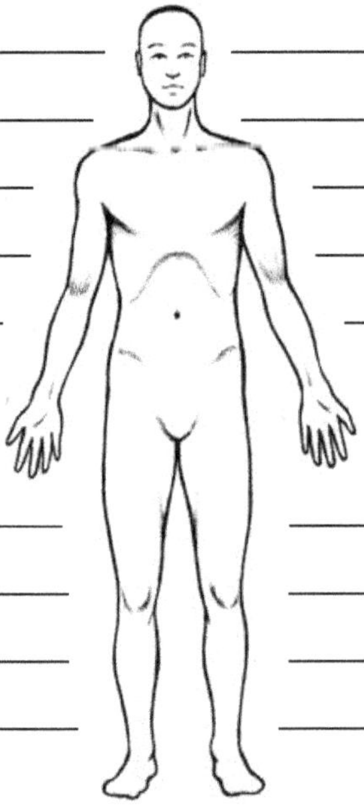

ENJOY THE JOURNEY ♥ ENJOY THE JOURNEY

ENJOY THE JOURNEY ♥ ENJOY THE JOURNEY ♥

ENJOY THE JOURNEY ♥ ENJOY THE JOURNEY ♥ ENJOY THE JOURNEY

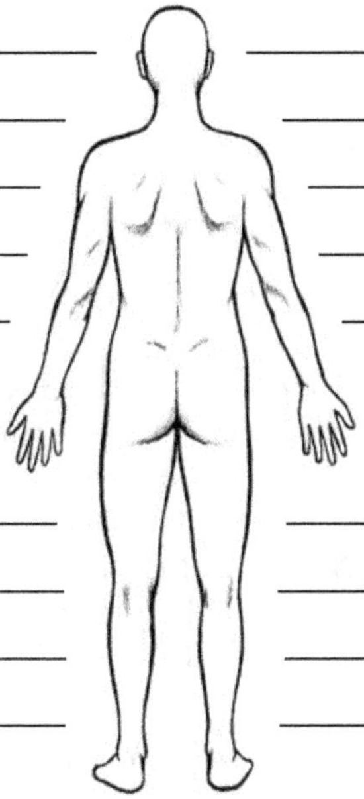

ENJOY THE JOURNEY ♥ ENJOY THE JOURNEY ♥

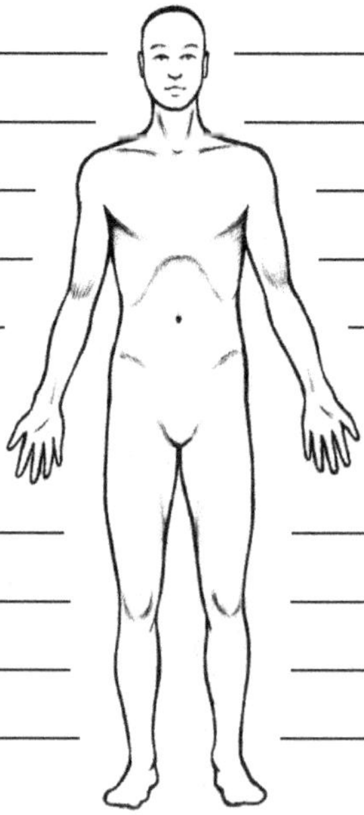

ASK YOURSELF QUESTIONS ♥ ASK YOURSELF QUESTIONS

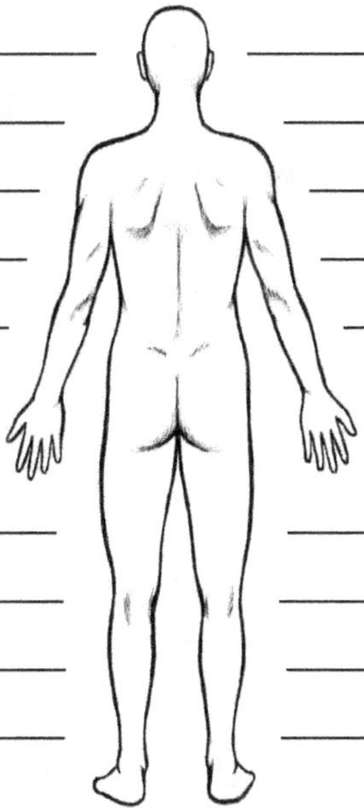

ASK YOURSELF QUESTIONS ♥ ASK YOURSELF QUESTIONS

SEEK THE ANSWER WITHIN ♥ SEEK THE ANSWER WITHIN

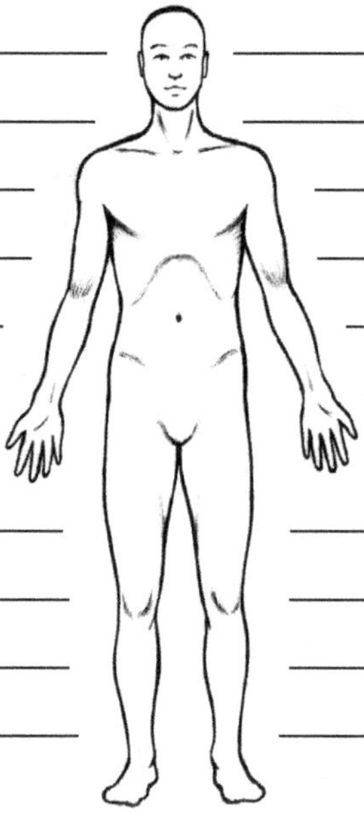

SEEK THE ANSWER WITHIN ♥ SEEK THE ANSWER WITHIN

SEEK THE ANSWER WITHIN ♥ SEEK THE ANSWER WITHIN

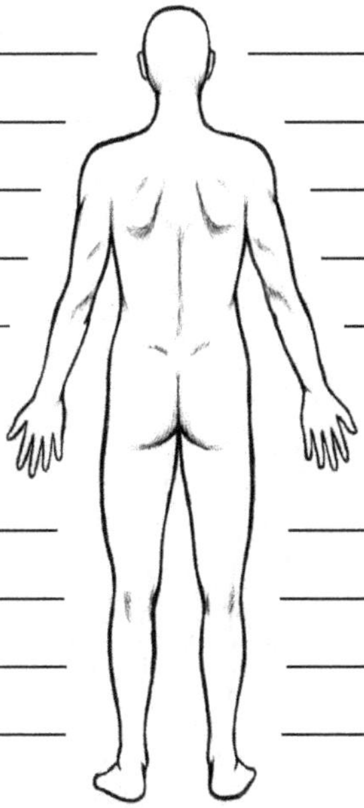

SEEK THE ANSWER WITHIN ♥ SEEK THE ANSWER WITHIN ♥

FEET: FOUNDATION ♥ FEET: FOUNDATION ♥ FEET: FOUNDATION

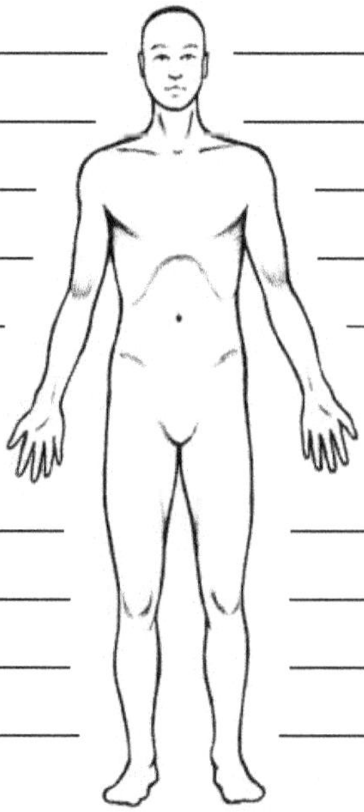

FEET: FOUNDATION ♥ FEET: FOUNDATION ♥ FEET: FOUNDATION

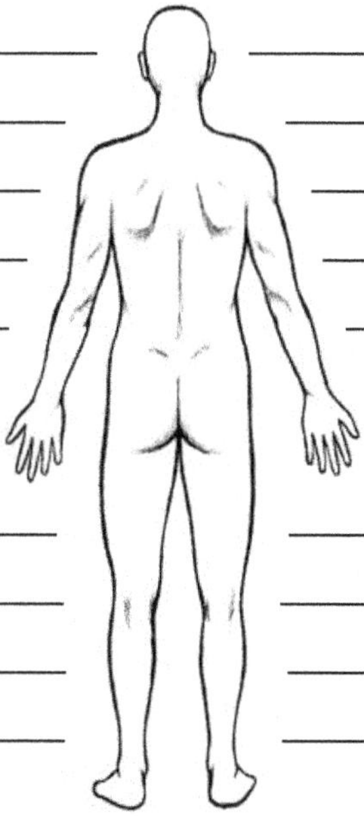

BE CURIOUS ♥ BE CURIOUS

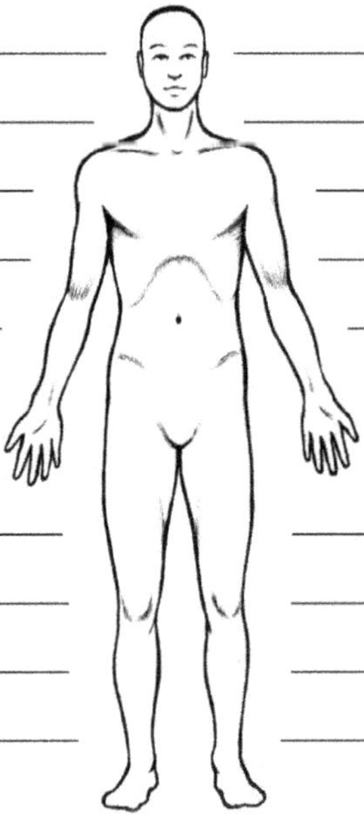

BE CURIOUS ♥ BE CURIOUS

BE CURIOUS ❤ BE CURIOUS ❤

BE CURIOUS ❤ BE CURIOUS ❤ BE CURIOUS

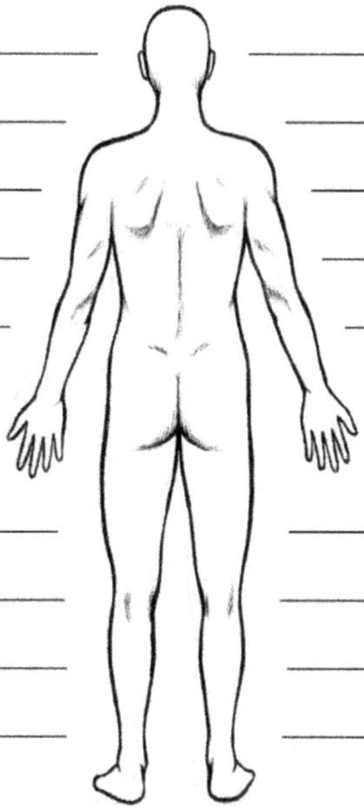

BE CURIOUS ❤ BE CURIOUS ❤

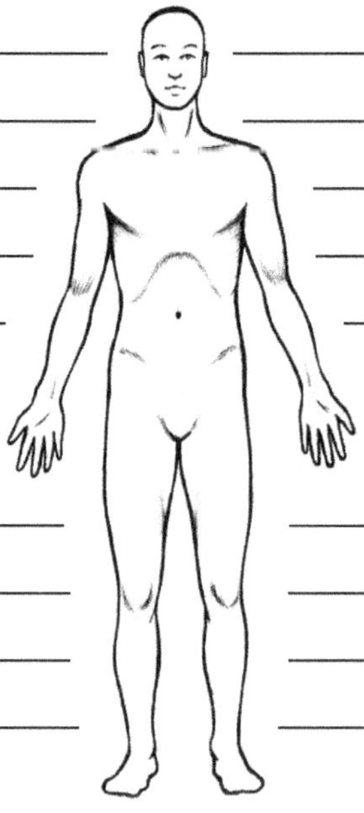

JOINTS: ARTICULATE MOVEMENT JOINTS: ARTICULATE MOVEMENT

JOINTS: ARTICULATE MOVEMENT JOINTS: ARTICULATE MOVEMENT

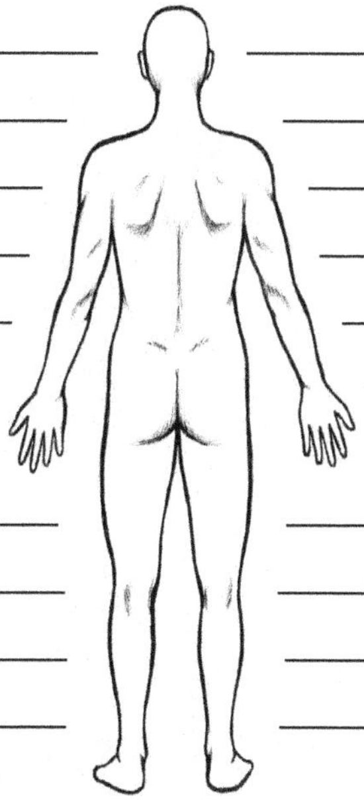

MOVE INTO YOURSELF ♥ MOVE INTO YOURSELF

MOVE INTO YOURSELF ♥ MOVE INTO YOURSELF ♥ MOVE INTO YOURSELF

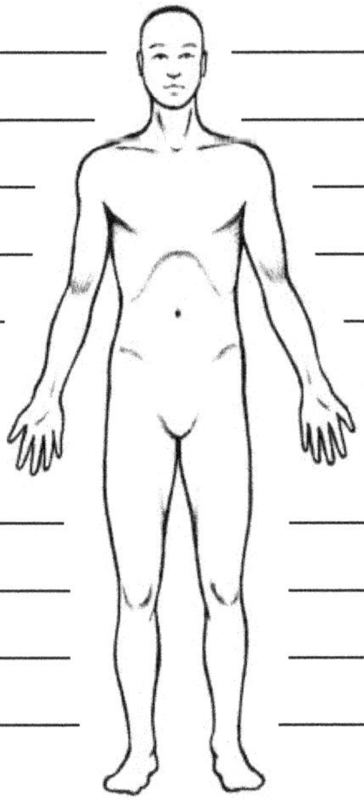

MOVE INTO YOURSELF ♥ MOVE INTO YOURSELF

MOVE INTO YOURSELF ♥ MOVE INTO YOURSELF ♥ MOVE INTO YOURSELF

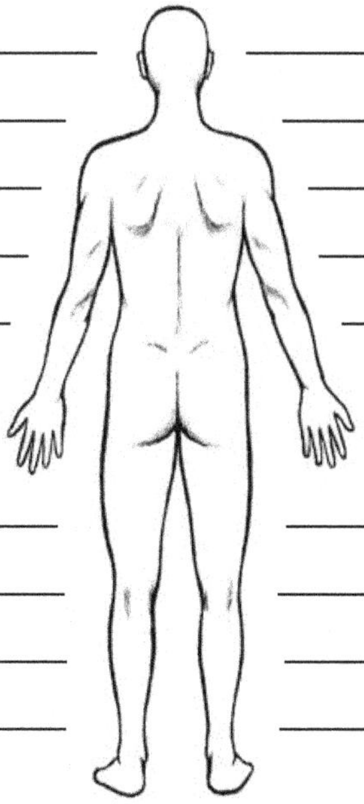

LEGS: HOW YOU STAND & MOVE ♥ LEGS: HOW YOU STAND & MOVE

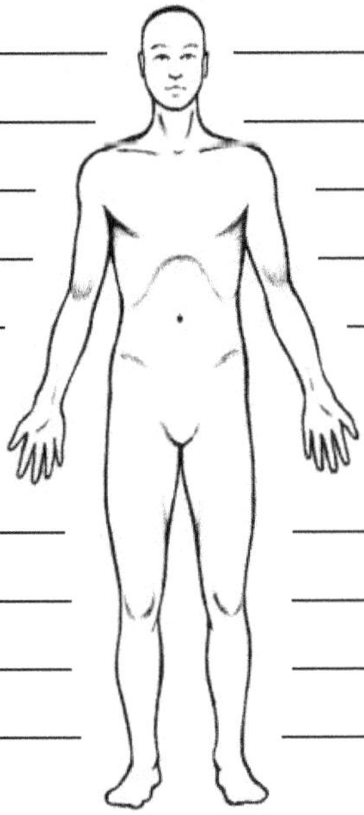

LEGS: HOW YOU STAND & MOVE ♥ LEGS: HOW YOU STAND & MOVE

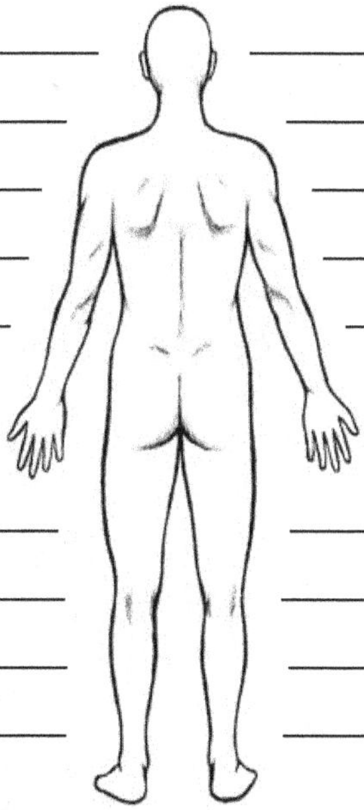

FOLLOW THE FEELINGS ♥ FOLLOW THE FEELINGS

FOLLOW THE FEELINGS ♥ FOLLOW THE FEELINGS

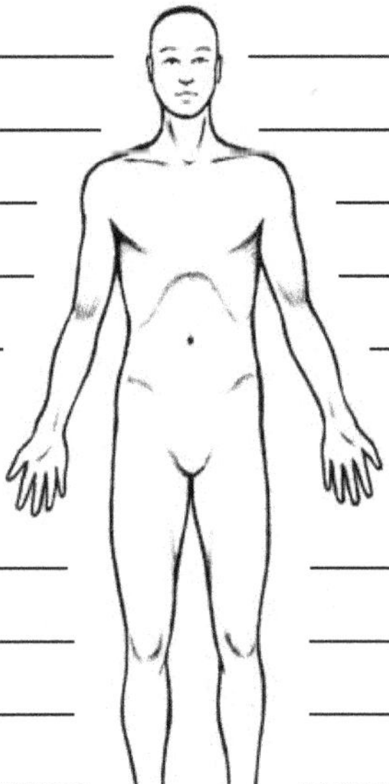

FOLLOW THE FEELINGS ♥ FOLLOW THE FEELINGS

FOLLOW THE FEELINGS ♥ FOLLOW THE FEELINGS

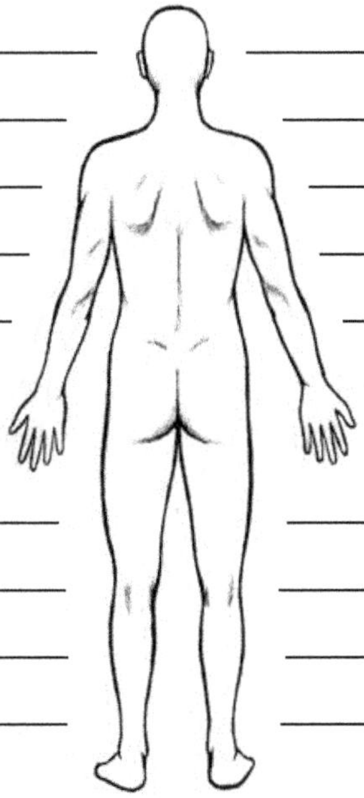

FOLLOW THE FEELINGS ♥ FOLLOW THE FEELINGS ♥

PELVIS: CREATIVE LIFE FORCE ♥ PELVIS: CREATIVE LIFE FORCE

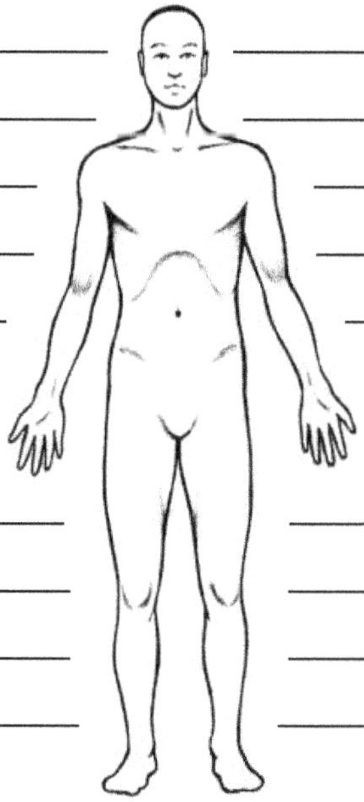

PELVIS: CREATIVE LIFE FORCE ♥ PELVIS: CREATIVE LIFE FORCE

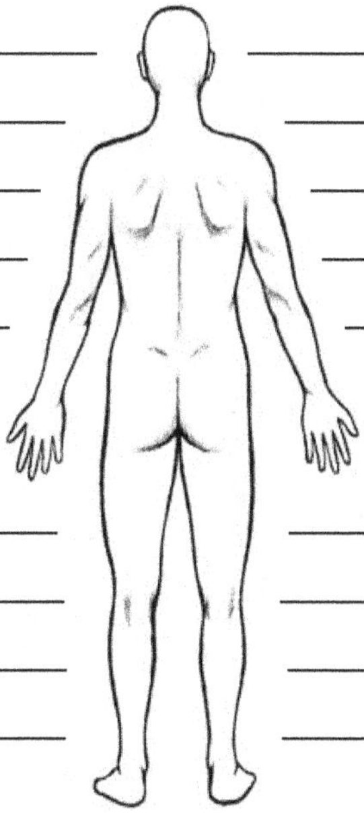

EXPLORE THE EXPERIENCE ♥ EXPLORE THE EXPERIENCE

EXPLORE THE EXPERIENCE ♥ EXPLORE THE EXPERIENCE

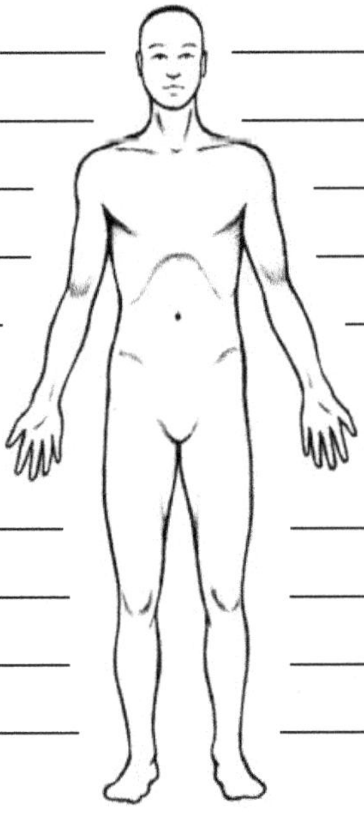

EXPLORE THE EXPERIENCE ♥ EXPLORE THE EXPERIENCE

EXPLORE THE EXPERIENCE ♥ EXPLORE THE EXPERIENCE

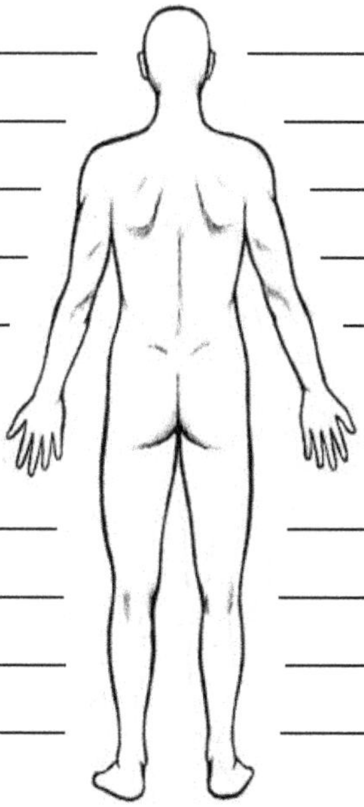

BELLY: EMOTIONAL CENTER ♥ BELLY: EMOTIONAL CENTER ♥ BELLY: EMOTIONAL CENTER

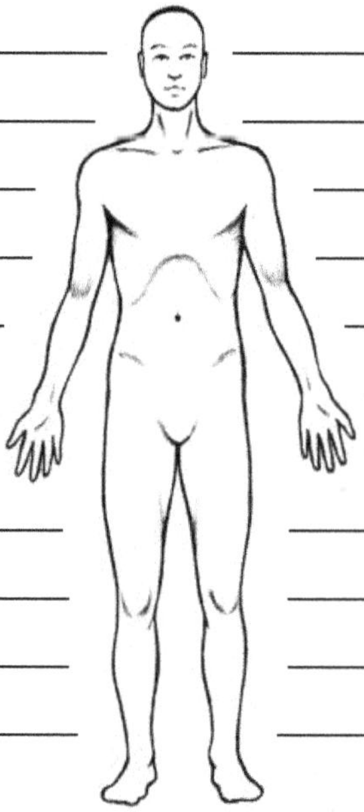

BELLY: EMOTIONAL CENTER ♥ BELLY: EMOTIONAL CENTER ♥ BELLY: EMOTIONAL CENTER

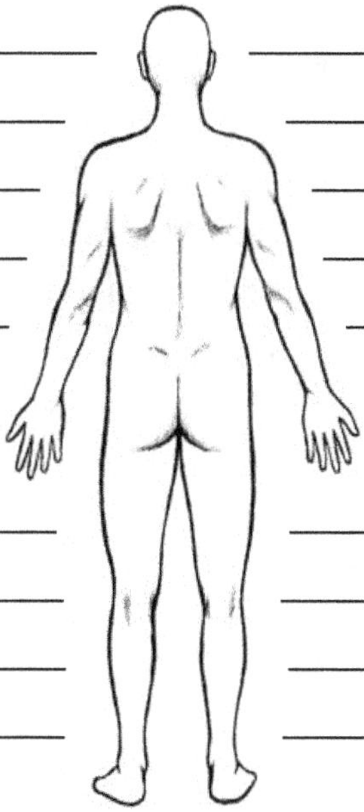

ANSWER TO YOUR FEELINGS ♥ ANSWER TO YOUR FEELINGS

ANSWER TO YOUR FEELINGS ♥ ANSWER TO YOUR FEELINGS

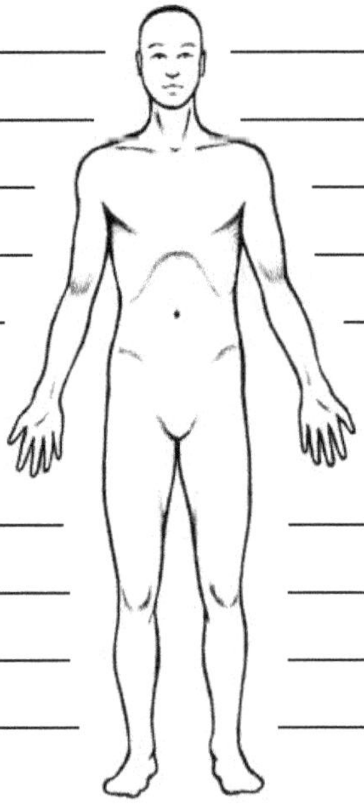

ANSWER TO YOUR FEELINGS ♥ ANSWER TO YOUR FEELINGS

ANSWER TO YOUR FEELINGS ♥ ANSWER TO YOUR FEELINGS

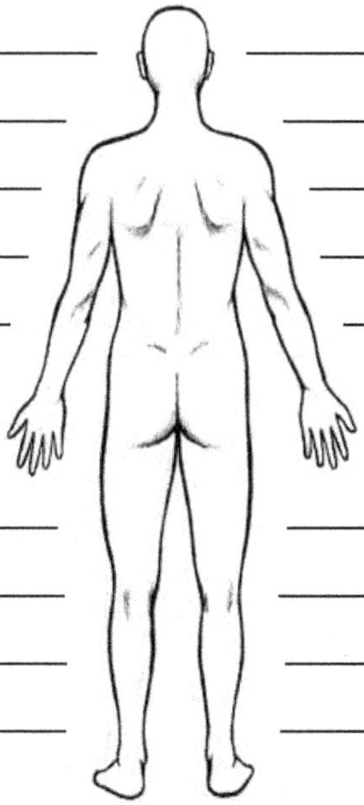

ANSWER TO YOUR FEELINGS ♥ ANSWER TO YOUR FEELINGS ♥

CHEST: HEART CENTER ❤ CHEST: HEART CENTER ❤ CHEST: HEART CENTER

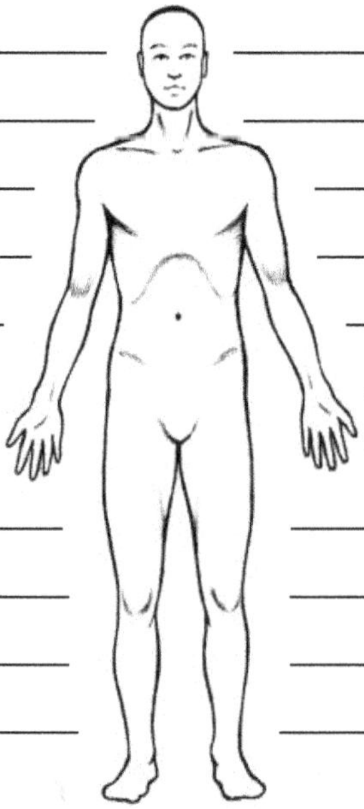

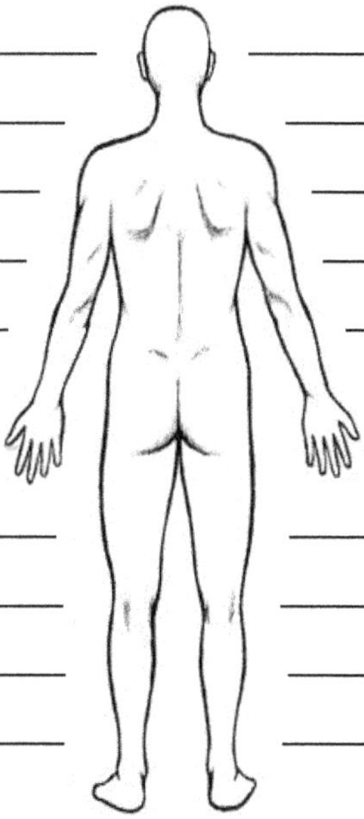

CHEST: HEART CENTER ♥ CHEST: HEART CENTER ♥ CHEST: HEART CENTER

LEAD WITH YOUR HEART ♥ LEAD WITH YOUR HEART

LEAD WITH YOUR HEART ♥ LEAD WITH YOUR HEART

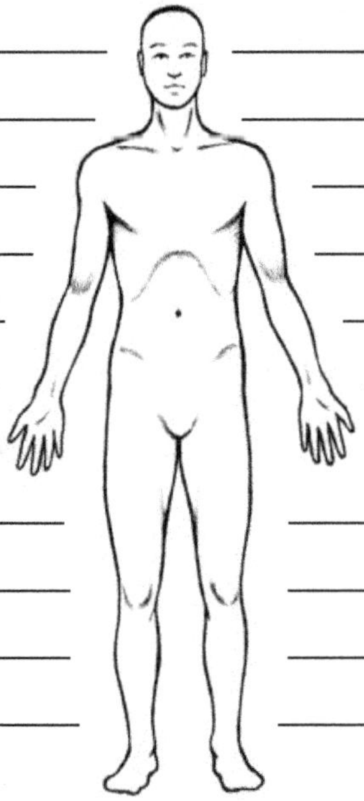

LEAD WITH YOUR HEART ♥ LEAD WITH YOUR HEART

LEAD WITH YOUR HEART ♥ LEAD WITH YOUR HEART ♥

LEAD WITH YOUR HEART ♥ LEAD WITH YOUR HEART

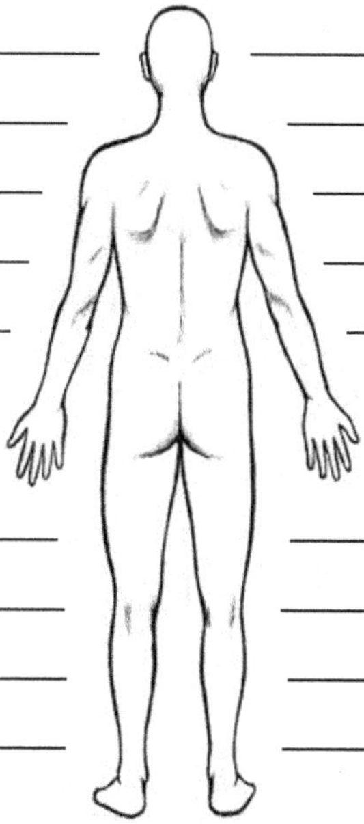

LEAD WITH YOUR HEART ♥ LEAD WITH YOUR HEART ♥

RIBS: HEART SUPPORT ❤ RIBS: HEART SUPPORT ❤ RIBS: HEART SUPPORT

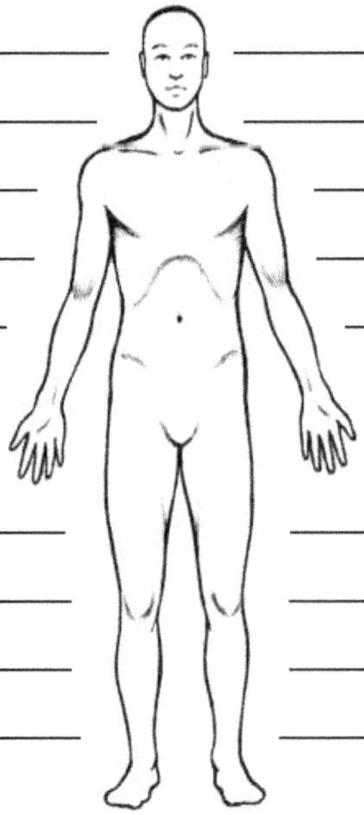

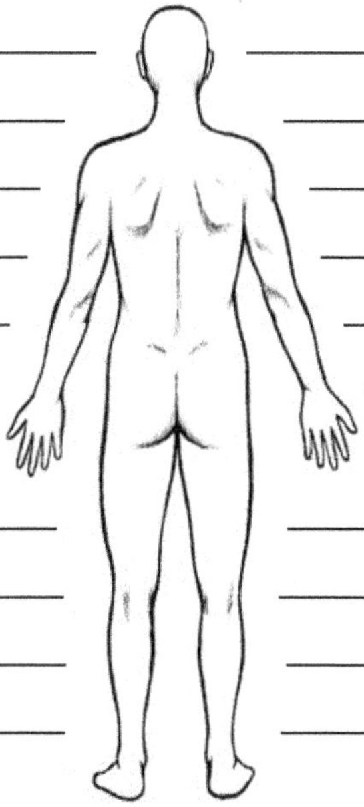

RIBS: HEART SUPPORT ♥ RIBS: HEART SUPPORT ♥ RIBS: HEART SUPPORT

TRUST YOUR HEART ♥ TRUST YOUR HEART ♥ TRUST YOUR HEART

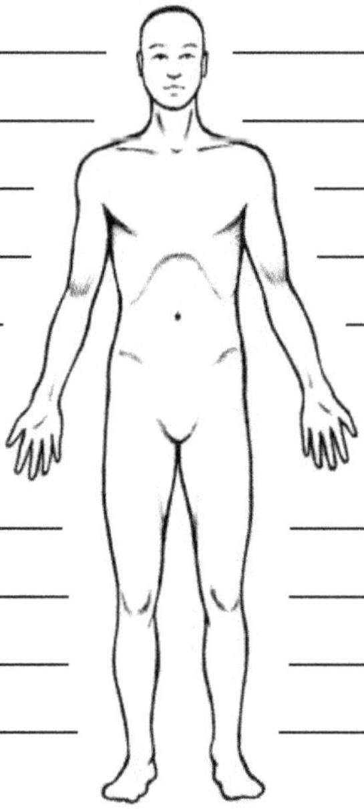

TRUST YOUR HEART ♥ TRUST YOUR HEART

TRUST YOUR HEART ♥ TRUST YOUR HEART ♥

TRUST YOUR HEART ♥ TRUST YOUR HEART ♥ TRUST YOUR HEART

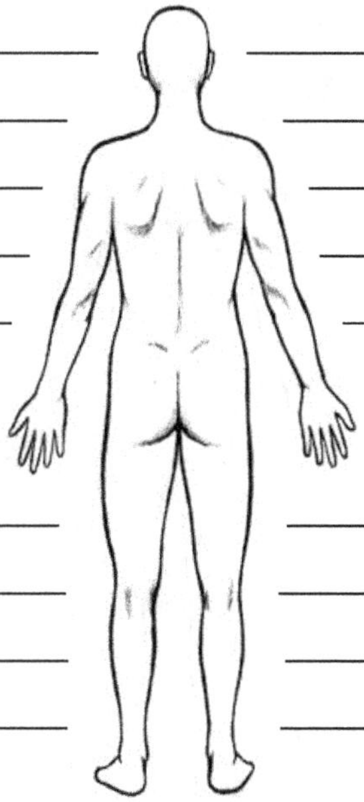

TRUST YOUR HEART ♥ TRUST YOUR HEART ♥

SHOULDERS: RESPONSIBILITY

SHOULDERS: RESPONSIBILITY
SHOULDERS: RESPONSIBILITY
SHOULDERS: RESPONSIBILITY

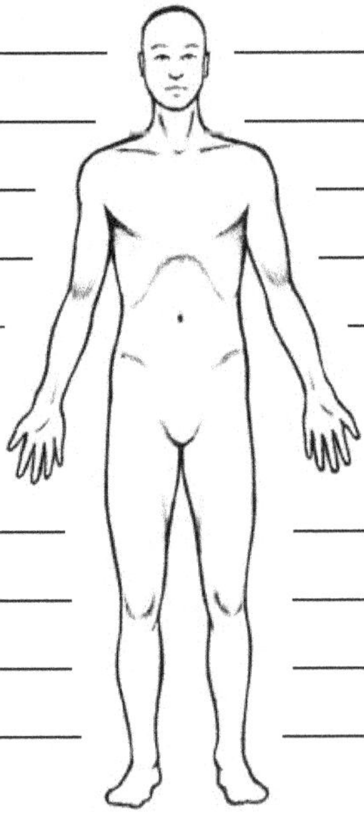

SHOULDERS: RESPONSIBILITY
SHOULDERS: RESPONSIBILITY

SHOULDERS: RESPONSIBILITY ♥ SHOULDERS: RESPONSIBILITY

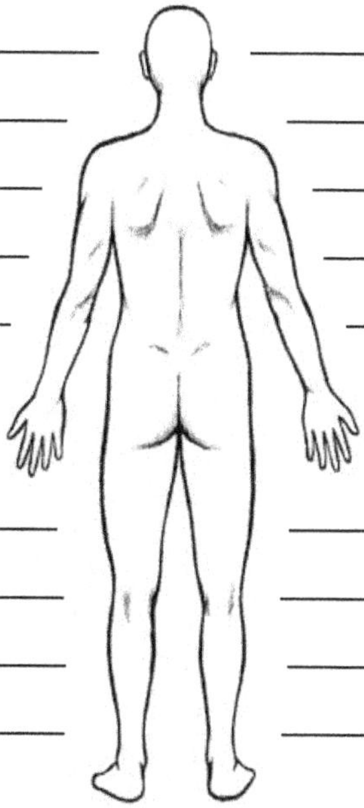

RESPONSE-ABILITY ♥ RESPONSE-ABILITY

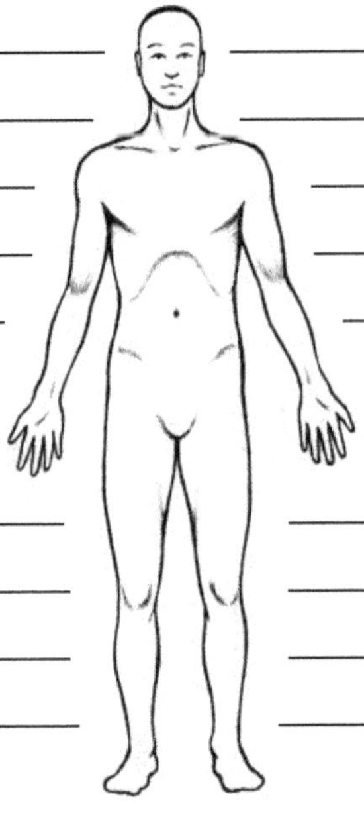

RESPONSE-ABILITY ♥ RESPONSE-ABILITY

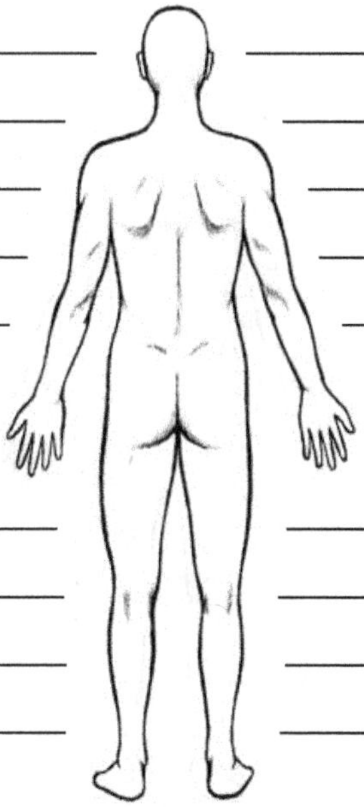

ARMS: EMBRACE ♥ ARMS: EMBRACE

ARMS: EMBRACE ♥ ARMS: EMBRACE ♥ ARMS: EMBRACE

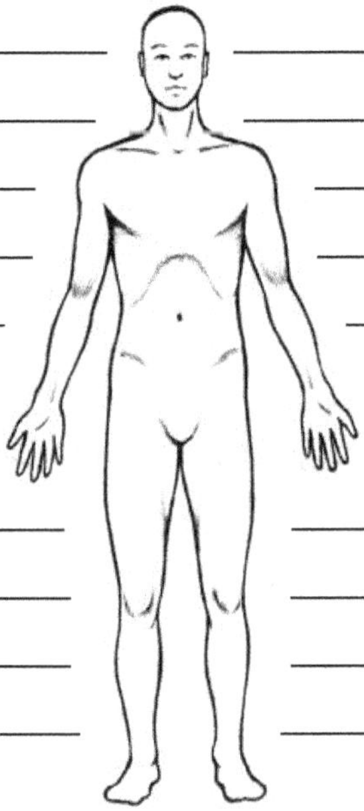

ARMS: EMBRACE ♥ ARMS: EMBRACE

ARMS: EMBRACE ❤ ARMS: EMBRACE ❤ ARMS: EMBRACE

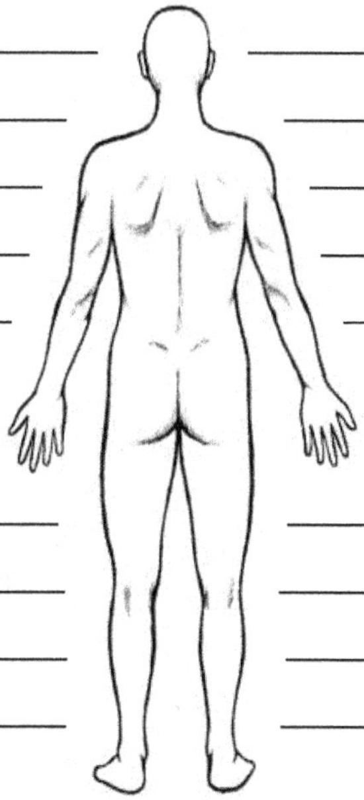

EMBRACE ALL THAT YOU FEEL ♥ EMBRACE ALL THAT YOU FEEL

EMBRACE ALL THAT YOU FEEL ♥ EMBRACE ALL THAT YOU FEEL

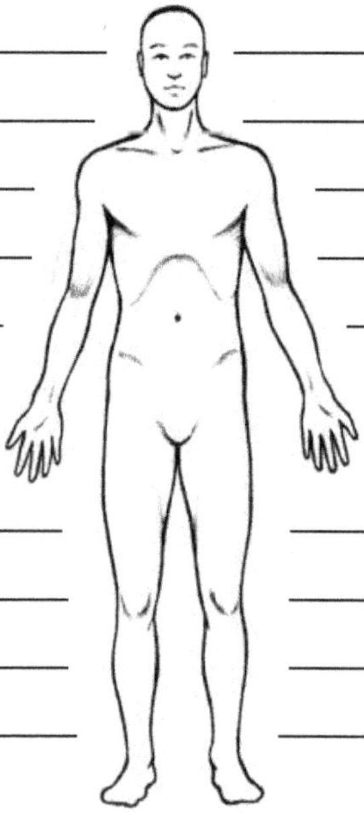

EMBRACE ALL THAT YOU FEEL ♥ EMBRACE ALL THAT YOU FEEL

EMBRACE ALL THAT YOU FEEL ♥ EMBRACE ALL THAT YOU FEEL ♥

EMBRACE ALL THAT YOU FEEL ♥ EMBRACE ALL THAT YOU FEEL

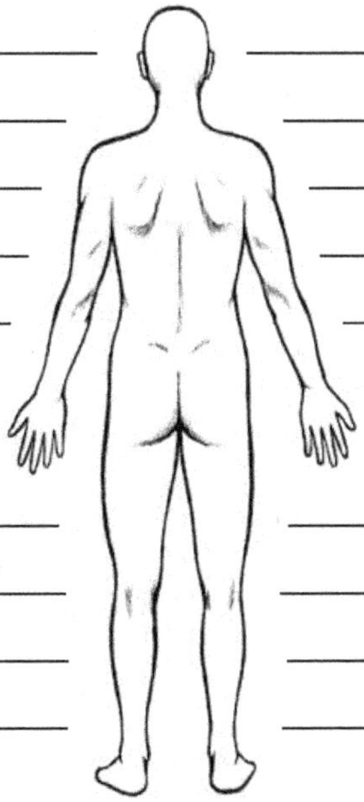

EMBRACE ALL THAT YOU FEEL ♥ EMBRACE ALL THAT YOU FEEL ♥

 HANDS: GIVE & RECEIVE

HANDS: GIVE & RECEIVE ♥ HANDS: GIVE & RECEIVE ♥ HANDS: GIVE & RECEIVE

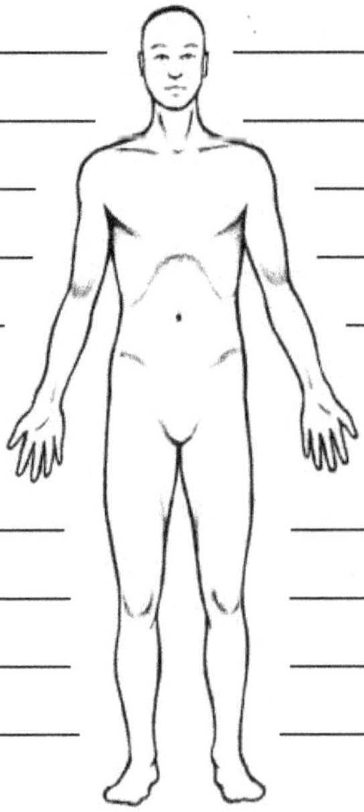

 HANDS: GIVE & RECEIVE

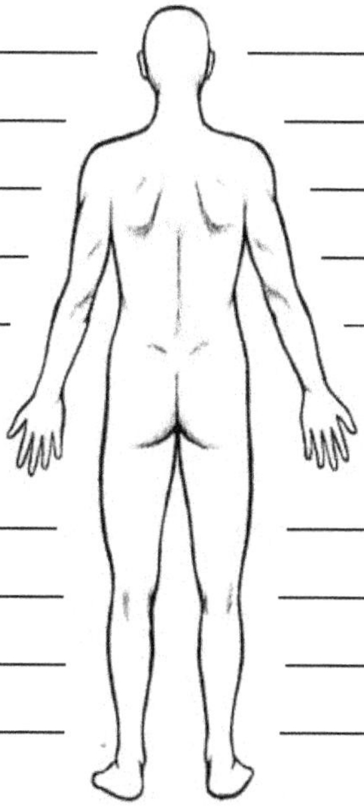

GIVING IS RECEIVING ♥ RECEIVING IS GIVING

RECEIVING IS GIVING

GIVING IS RECEIVING

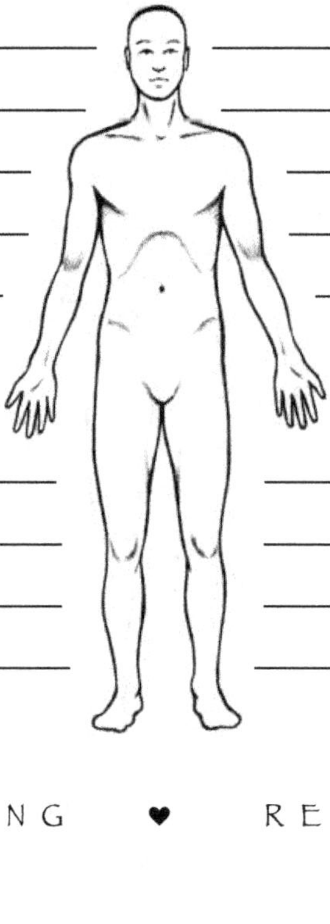

GIVING IS RECEIVING ♥ RECEIVING IS GIVING

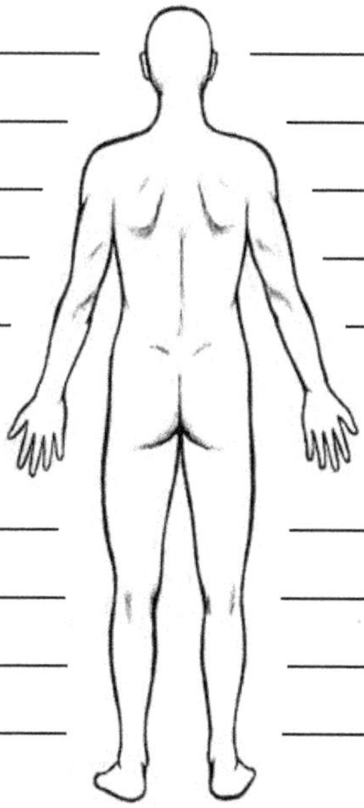

NECK: PATH OF COMMUNICATION BETWEEN HEAD & HEART

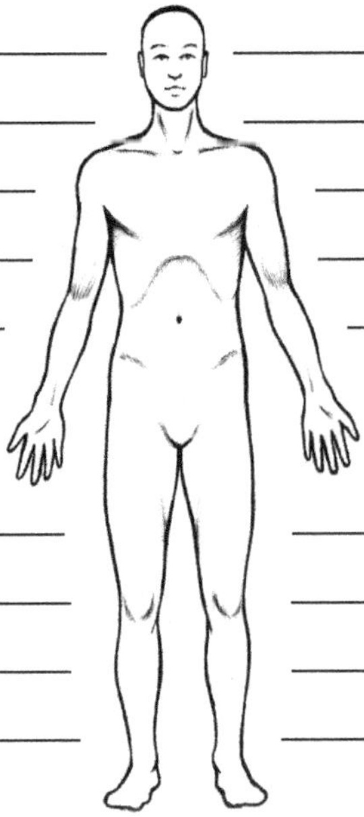

NECK: PATH OF COMMUNICATION BETWEEN HEAD & HEART

NECK: PATH OF COMMUNICATION BETWEEN HEAD & HEART

NECK: PATH OF COMMUNICATION BETWEEN HEAD & HEART

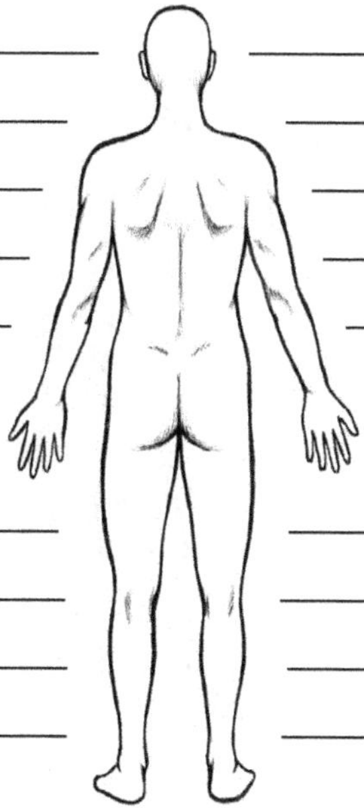

NECK: PATH OF COMMUNICATION BETWEEN HEAD & HEART

SPEAK THE WISDOM OF YOUR HEART ♥ SPEAK THE WISDOM OF YOUR HEART

SPEAK THE WISDOM OF YOUR HEART ♥ SPEAK THE WISDOM OF YOUR HEART

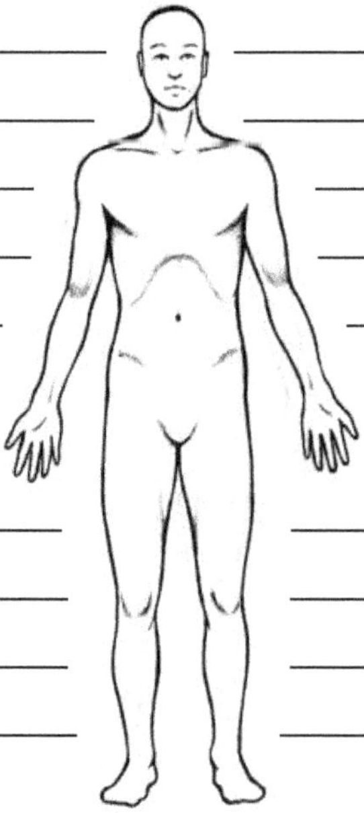

SPEAK THE WISDOM OF YOUR HEART ♥ SPEAK THE WISDOM OF YOUR HEART

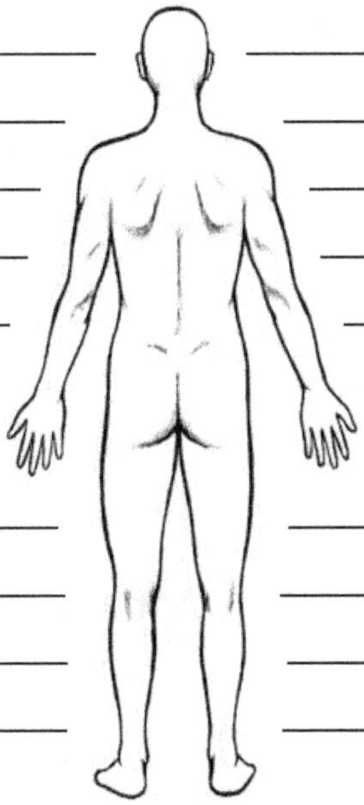

HEAD: WHERE YOU HOLD YOUR THOUGHTS

HEAD: WHERE YOU HOLD YOUR THOUGHTS
HEAD: WHERE YOU HOLD YOUR THOUGHTS
HEAD: WHERE YOU HOLD YOUR THOUGHTS
HEAD: WHERE YOU HOLD YOUR THOUGHTS
HEAD: WHERE YOU HOLD YOUR THOUGHTS

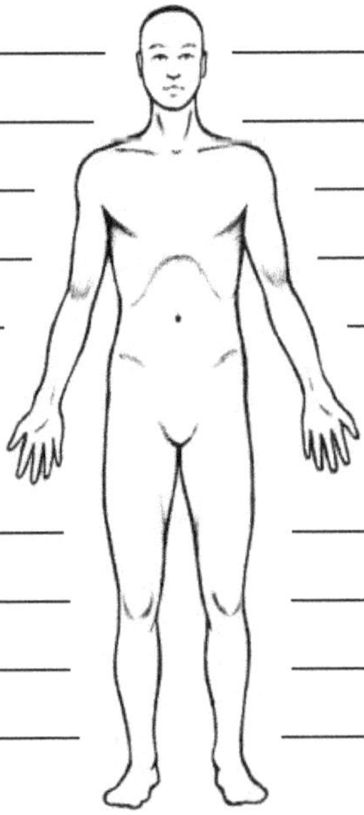

HEAD: WHERE YOU HOLD YOUR THOUGHTS ♥ HEAD: WHERE YOU HOLD YOUR THOUGHTS

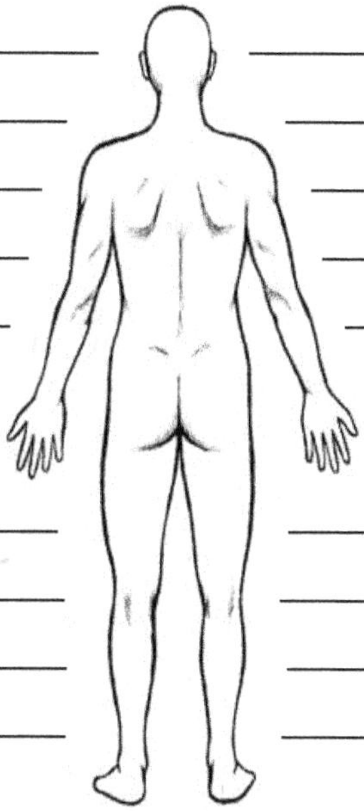

KNOW YOUR WISDOM ❤ KNOW YOUR WISDOM ❤ KNOW YOUR WISDOM

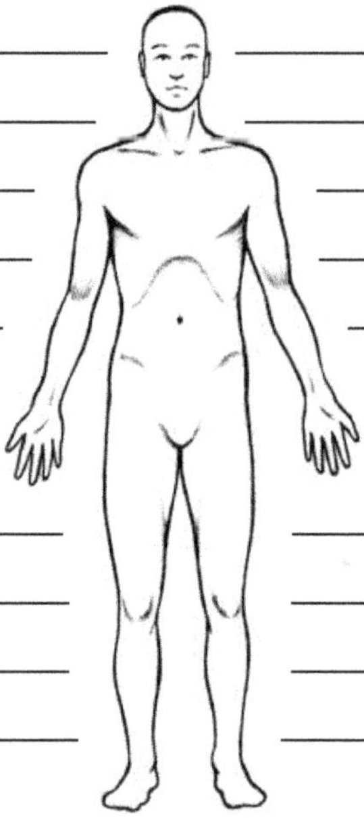

KNOW YOUR WISDOM ♥ KNOW YOUR WISDOM ♥ KNOW YOUR WISDOM

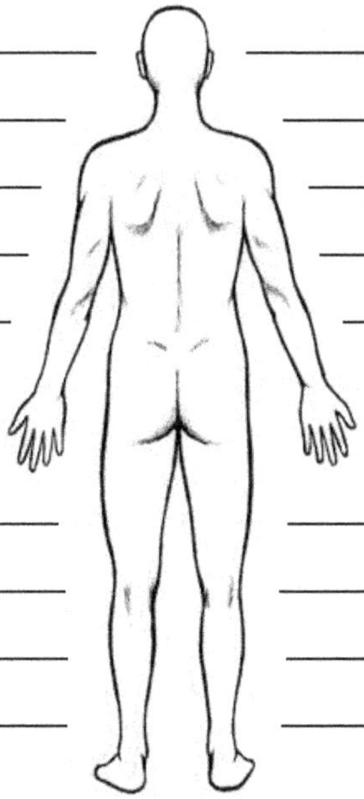

FACE: HOW YOU FACE THE WORLD ♥ FACE: HOW YOU FACE THE WORLD ♥ FACE: HOW YOU FACE THE WORLD

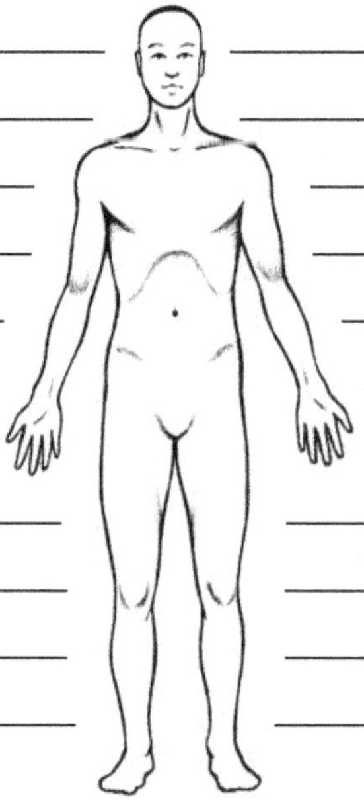

FACE: HOW YOU FACE THE WORLD ♥ FACE: HOW YOU FACE THE WORLD ♥ FACE: HOW YOU FACE THE WORLD

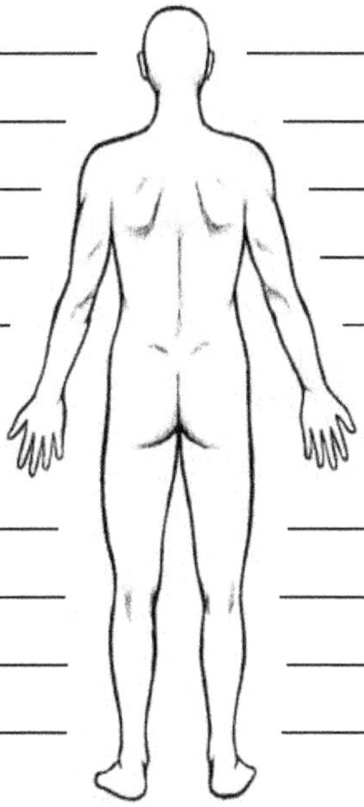

FACE THE WORLD FROM WITHIN ♥ FACE THE WORLD FROM WITHIN

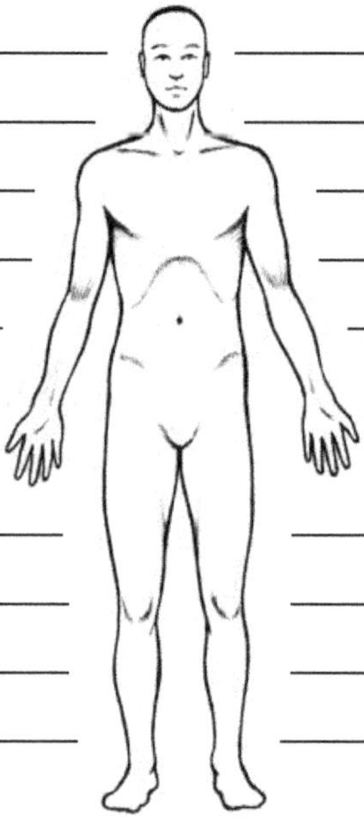

FACE THE WORLD FROM WITHIN ♥ FACE THE WORLD FROM WITHIN

FACE THE WORLD FROM WITHIN ♥ FACE THE WORLD FROM WITHIN ♥

FACE THE WORLD FROM WITHIN ♥ FACE THE WORLD FROM WITHIN

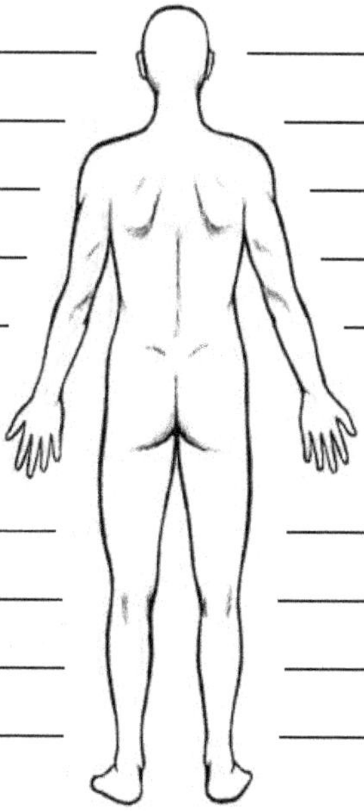

FACE THE WORLD FROM WITHIN ♥ FACE THE WORLD FROM WITHIN ♥

ENJOY THE JOURNEY ♥ ENJOY THE JOURNEY

ENJOY THE JOURNEY ♥ ENJOY THE JOURNEY ♥ ENJOY THE JOURNEY

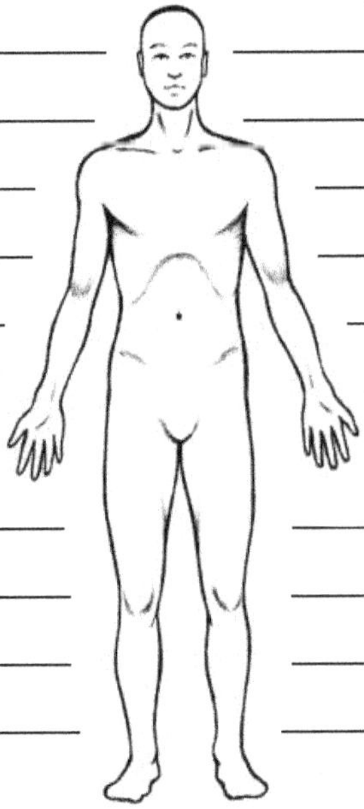

ENJOY THE JOURNEY ♥ ENJOY THE JOURNEY

ENJOY THE JOURNEY ♥ ENJOY THE JOURNEY ♥ ENJOY THE JOURNEY

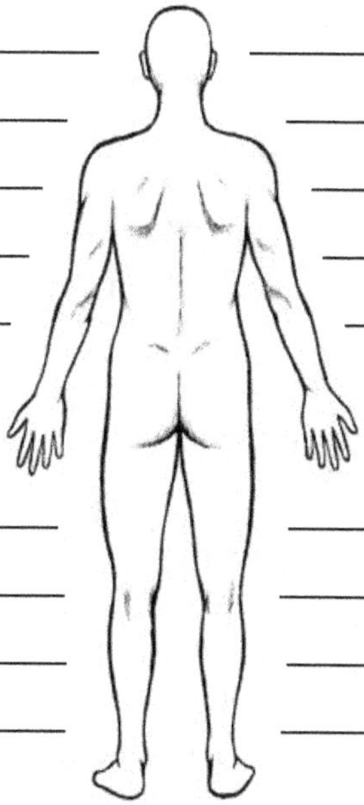

ASK YOURSELF QUESTIONS ♥ ASK YOURSELF QUESTIONS

ASK YOURSELF QUESTIONS ♥ ASK YOURSELF QUESTIONS

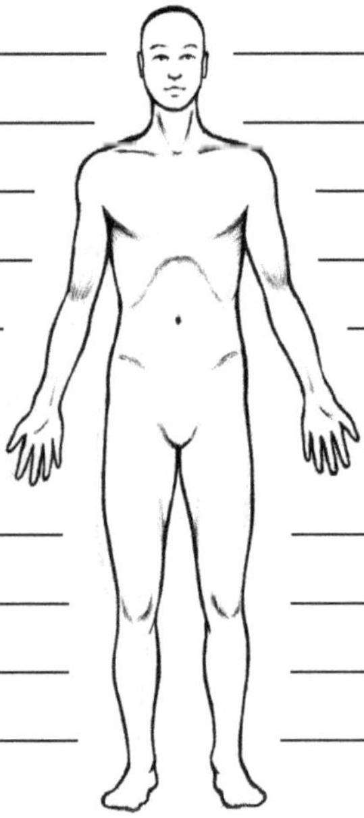

ASK YOURSELF QUESTIONS ♥ ASK YOURSELF QUESTIONS

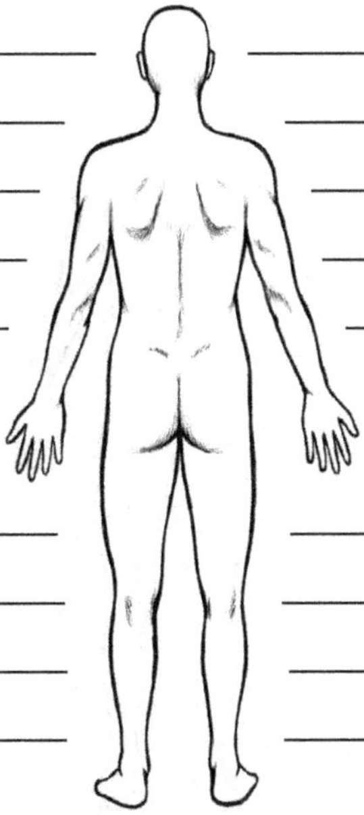

SEEK THE ANSWER WITHIN ♥ SEEK THE ANSWER WITHIN

SEEK THE ANSWER WITHIN ♥ SEEK THE ANSWER WITHIN

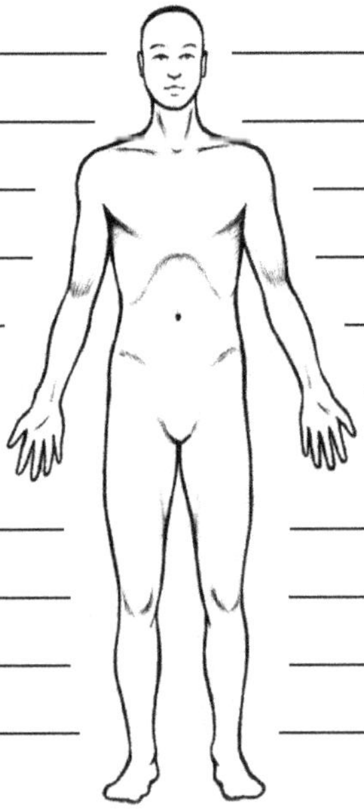

SEEK THE ANSWER WITHIN ♥ SEEK THE ANSWER WITHIN

SEEK THE ANSWER WITHIN ♥ SEEK THE ANSWER WITHIN ♥

SEEK THE ANSWER WITHIN ♥ SEEK THE ANSWER WITHIN

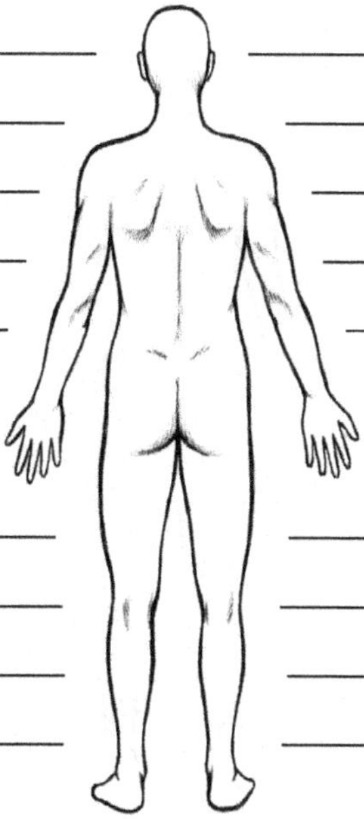

SEEK THE ANSWER WITHIN ♥ SEEK THE ANSWER WITHIN ♥

FEET: FOUNDATION ♥ FEET: FOUNDATION

FEET: FOUNDATION ♥ FEET: FOUNDATION ♥ FEET: FOUNDATION

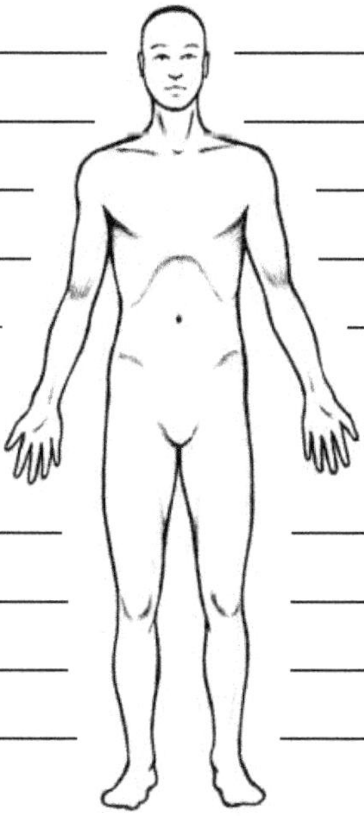

FEET: FOUNDATION ♥ FEET: FOUNDATION

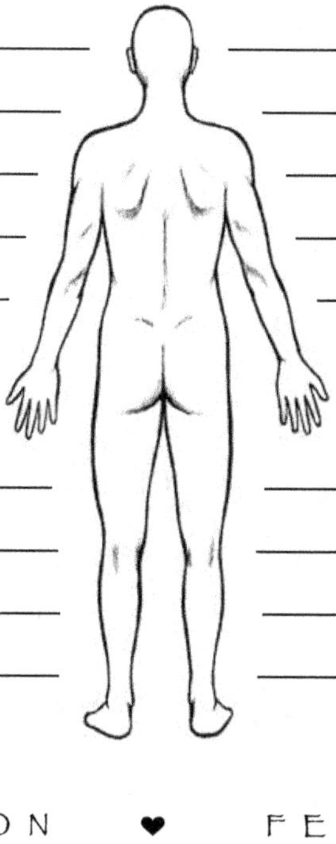

FEET: FOUNDATION ♥ FEET: FOUNDATION ♥ FEET: FOUNDATION

FEET: FOUNDATION ♥ FEET: FOUNDATION ♥

BE CURIOUS ♥ BE CURIOUS

BE CURIOUS ♥ BE CURIOUS ♥ BE CURIOUS

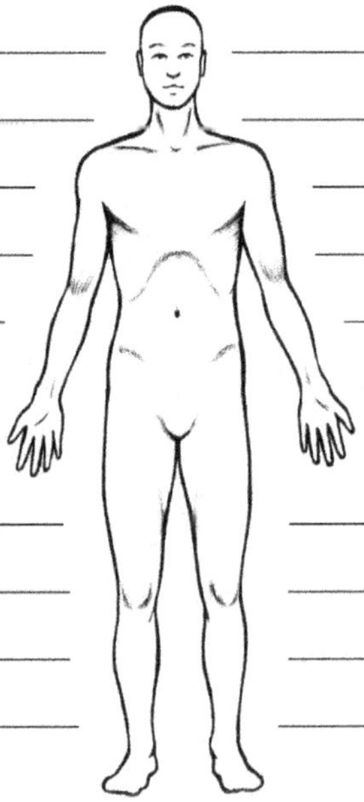

BE CURIOUS ♥ BE CURIOUS

BE CURIOUS ♥ BE CURIOUS ♥

BE CURIOUS ♥ BE CURIOUS ♥ BE CURIOUS

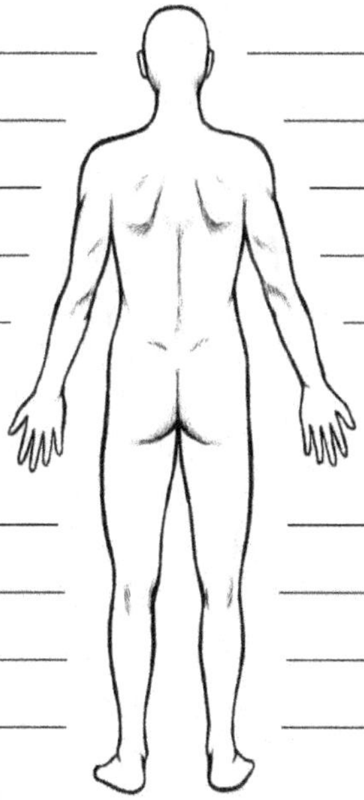

BE CURIOUS ♥ BE CURIOUS ♥

JOINTS: ARTICULATE MOVEMENT

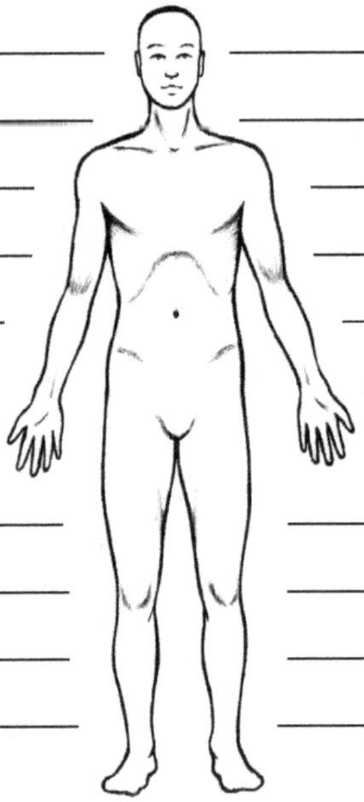

JOINTS: ARTICULATE MOVEMENT

JOINTS: ARTICULATE MOVEMENT

JOINTS: ARTICULATE MOVEMENT

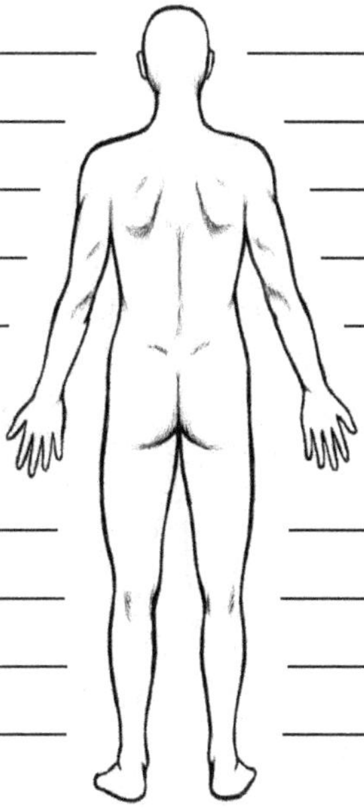

MOVE INTO YOURSELF ♥ MOVE INTO YOURSELF

MOVE INTO YOURSELF ♥ MOVE INTO YOURSELF ♥ MOVE INTO YOURSELF

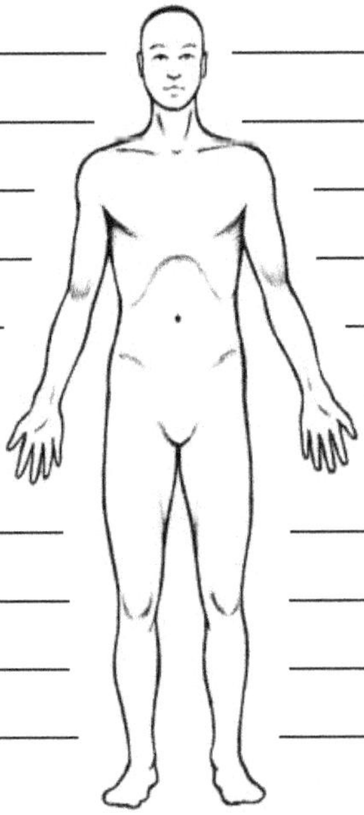

MOVE INTO YOURSELF ♥ MOVE INTO YOURSELF

MOVE INTO YOURSELF ♥ MOVE INTO YOURSELF ♥

MOVE INTO YOURSELF ♥ MOVE INTO YOURSELF ♥ MOVE INTO YOURSELF

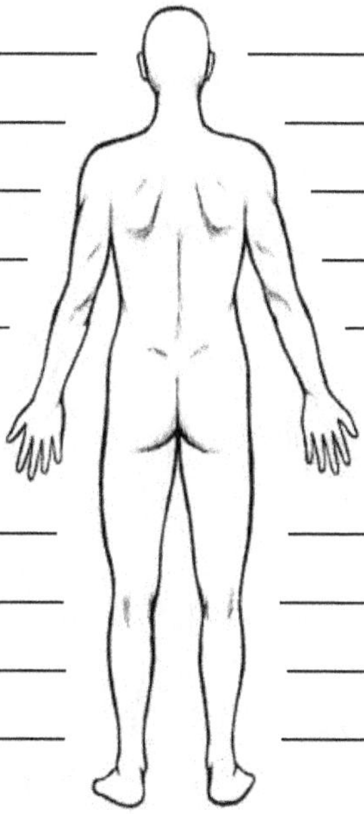

MOVE INTO YOURSELF ♥ MOVE INTO YOURSELF ♥

LEGS: HOW YOU STAND & MOVE ♥ LEGS: HOW YOU STAND & MOVE

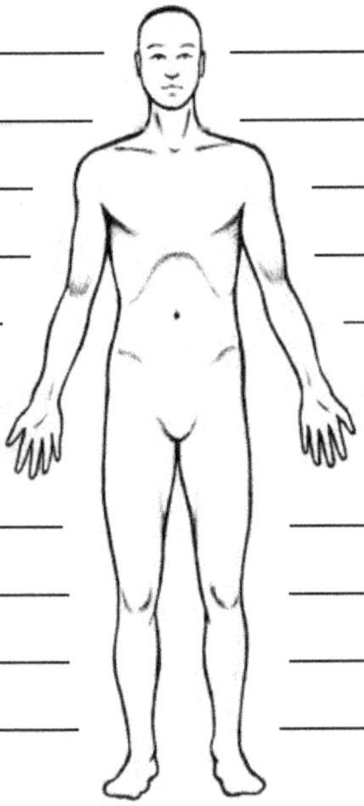

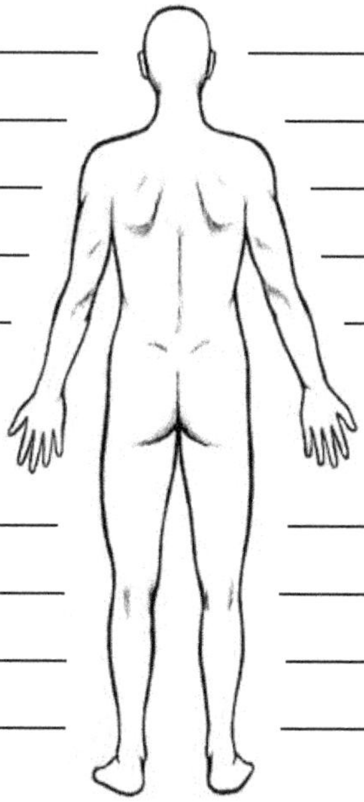

FOLLOW THE FEELINGS ♥ FOLLOW THE FEELINGS

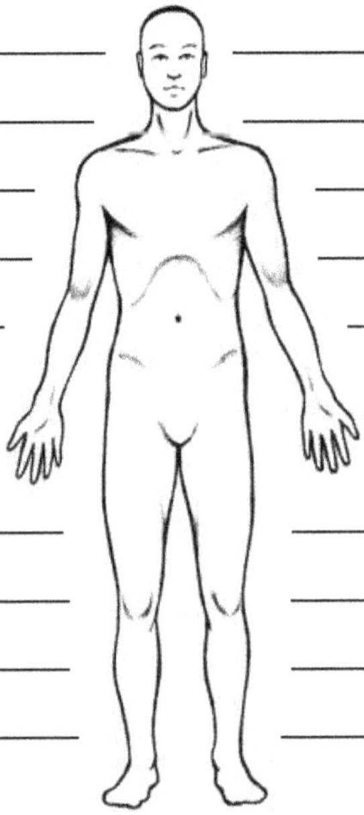

FOLLOW THE FEELINGS ♥ FOLLOW THE FEELINGS

FOLLOW THE FEELINGS ♥ FOLLOW THE FEELINGS ♥

FOLLOW THE FEELINGS ♥ FOLLOW THE FEELINGS

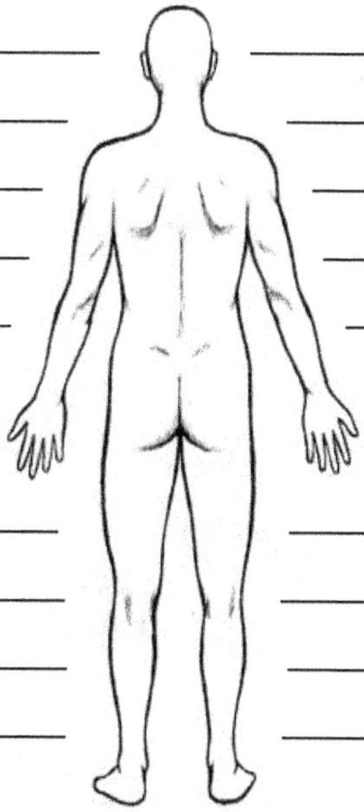

FOLLOW THE FEELINGS ♥ FOLLOW THE FEELINGS ♥

PELVIS: CREATIVE LIFE FORCE
PELVIS: CREATIVE LIFE FORCE
PELVIS: CREATIVE LIFE FORCE

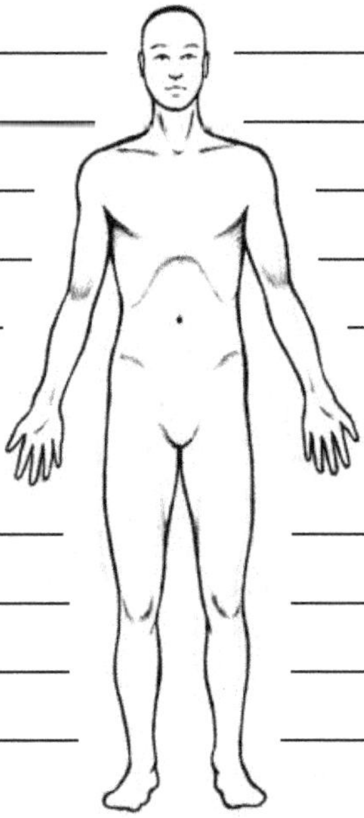

PELVIS: CREATIVE LIFE FORCE

PELVIS: CREATIVE LIFE FORCE ♥ PELVIS: CREATIVE LIFE FORCE

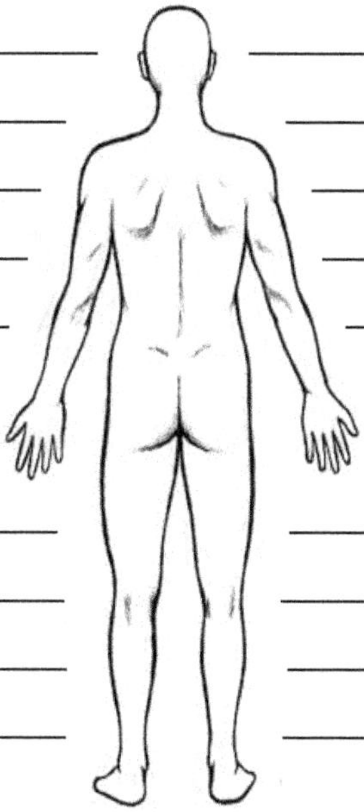

EXPLORE THE EXPERIENCE ♥ EXPLORE THE EXPERIENCE

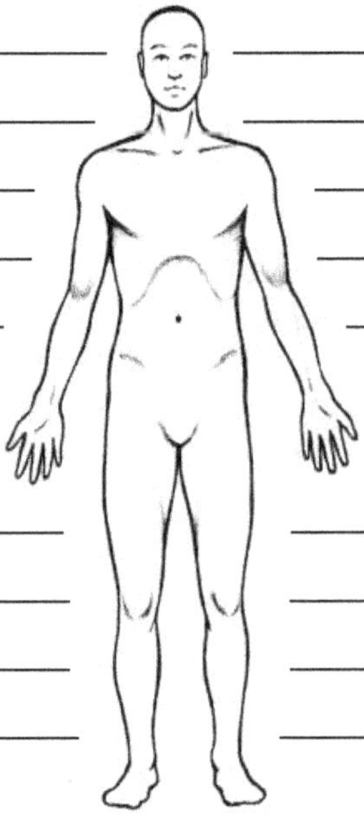

EXPLORE THE EXPERIENCE ♥ EXPLORE THE EXPERIENCE

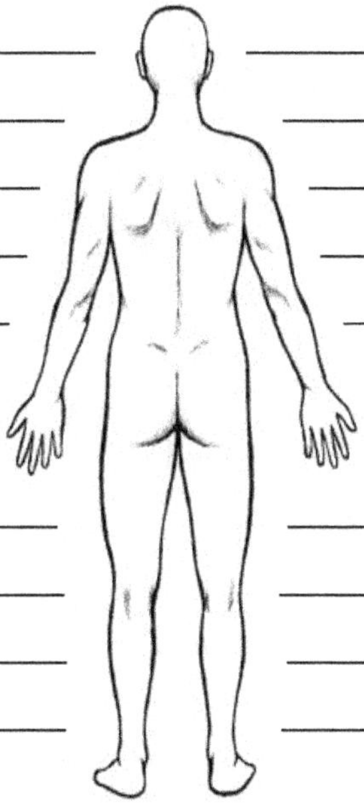

BELLY: EMOTIONAL CENTER ♥ BELLY: EMOTIONAL CENTER ♥ BELLY: EMOTIONAL CENTER

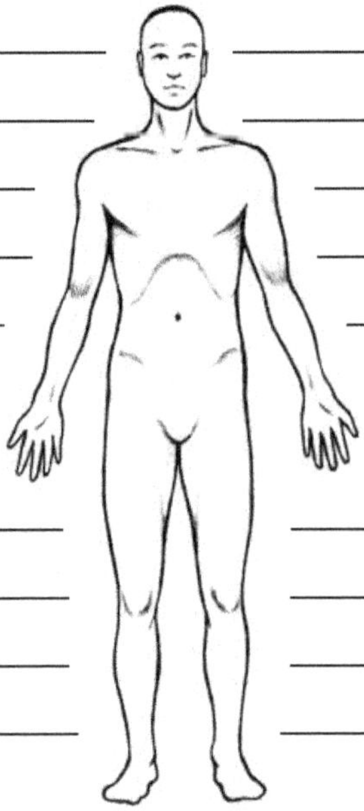

BELLY: EMOTIONAL CENTER ♥ BELLY: EMOTIONAL CENTER ♥ BELLY: EMOTIONAL CENTER

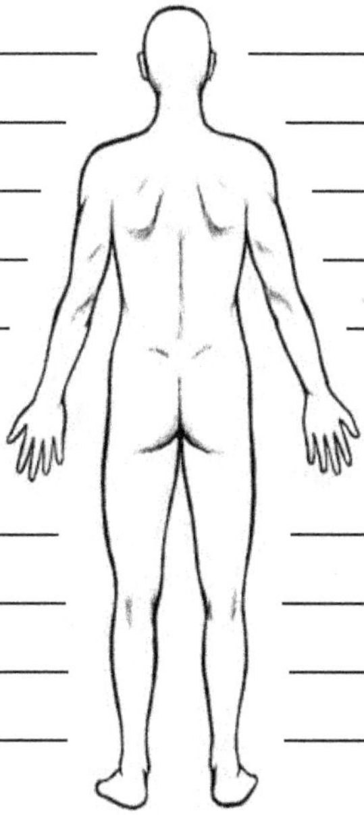

ANSWER TO YOUR FEELINGS ♥ ANSWER TO YOUR FEELINGS

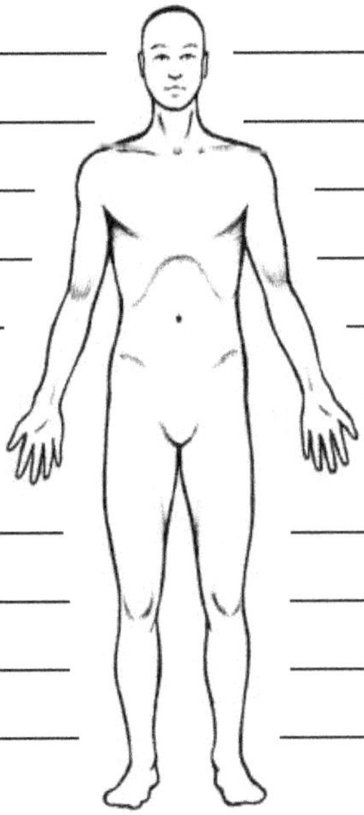

ANSWER TO YOUR FEELINGS ♥ ANSWER TO YOUR FEELINGS

ANSWER TO YOUR FEELINGS ♥ ANSWER TO YOUR FEELINGS ♥

ANSWER TO YOUR FEELINGS ♥ ANSWER TO YOUR FEELINGS

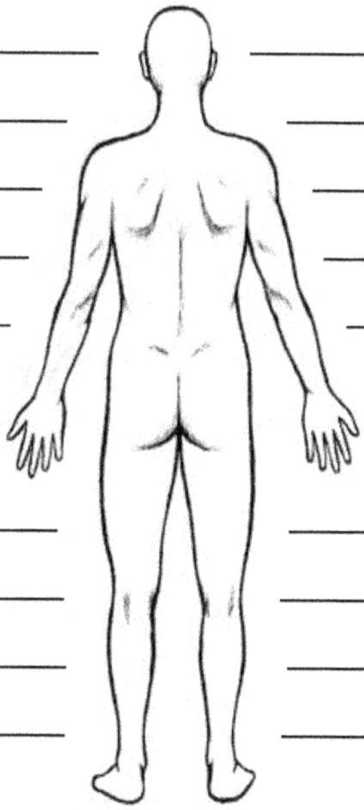

ANSWER TO YOUR FEELINGS ♥ ANSWER TO YOUR FEELINGS ♥

CHEST: HEART CENTER ❤ CHEST: HEART CENTER ❤ CHEST: HEART CENTER

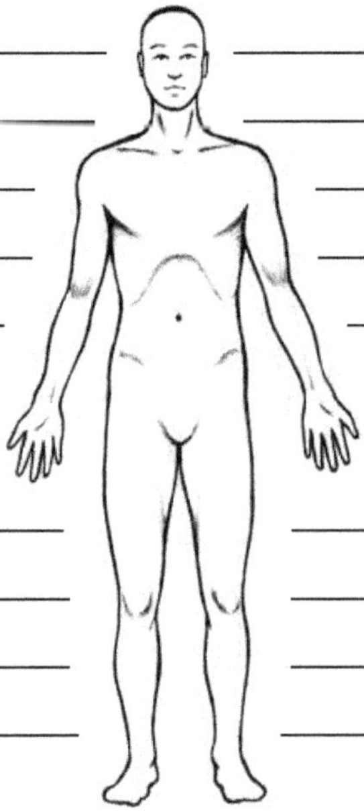

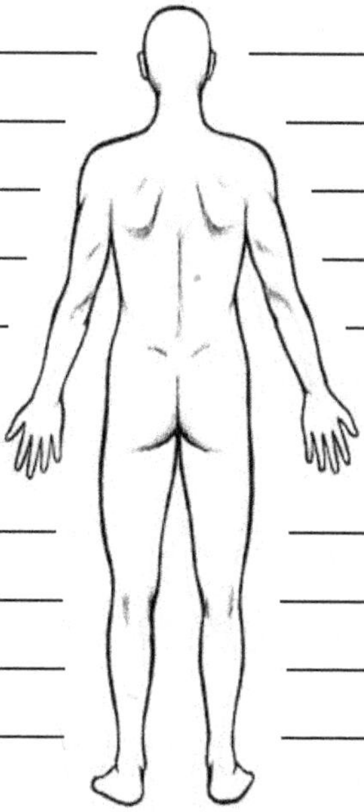

CHEST: HEART CENTER ♥ CHEST: HEART CENTER ♥ CHEST: HEART CENTER

CHEST: HEART CENTER ♥ CHEST: HEART CENTER ♥

LEAD WITH YOUR HEART ♥ LEAD WITH YOUR HEART

LEAD WITH YOUR HEART ♥ LEAD WITH YOUR HEART

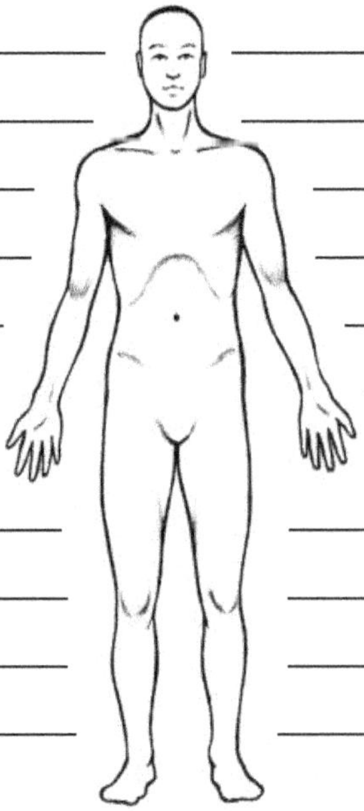

LEAD WITH YOUR HEART ♥ LEAD WITH YOUR HEART

LEAD WITH YOUR HEART ♥ LEAD WITH YOUR HEART

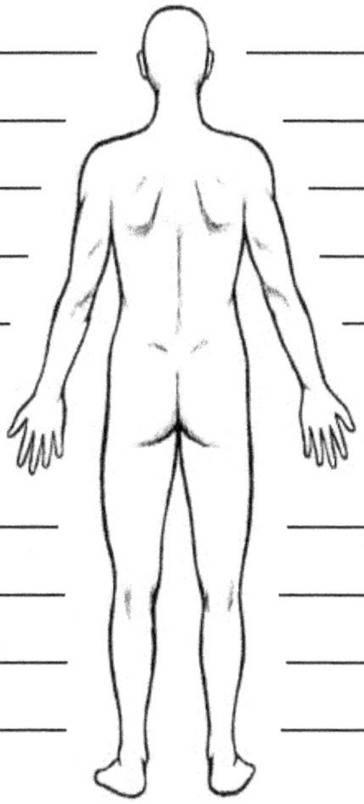

LEAD WITH YOUR HEART ♥ LEAD WITH YOUR HEART ♥

RIBS: HEART SUPPORT
RIBS: HEART SUPPORT
RIBS: HEART SUPPORT
RIBS: HEART SUPPORT

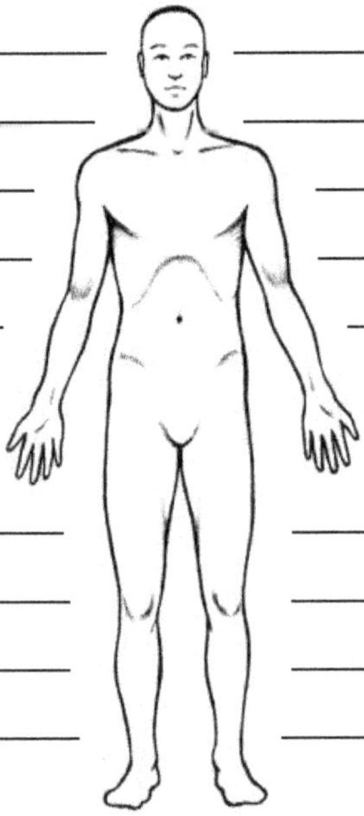

RIBS: HEART SUPPORT

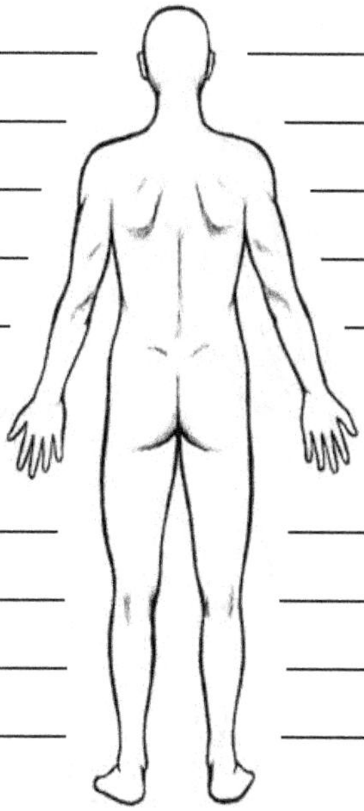

TRUST YOUR HEART ♥ TRUST YOUR HEART

TRUST YOUR HEART ♥ TRUST YOUR HEART ♥ TRUST YOUR HEART

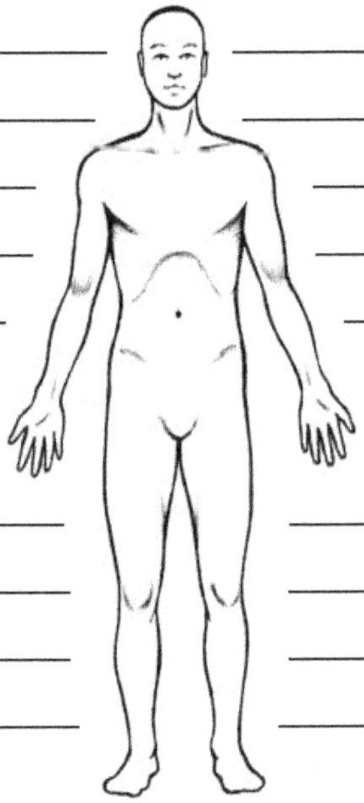

TRUST YOUR HEART ♥ TRUST YOUR HEART

TRUST YOUR HEART ♥ TRUST YOUR HEART ♥

TRUST YOUR HEART ♥ TRUST YOUR HEART ♥ TRUST YOUR HEART

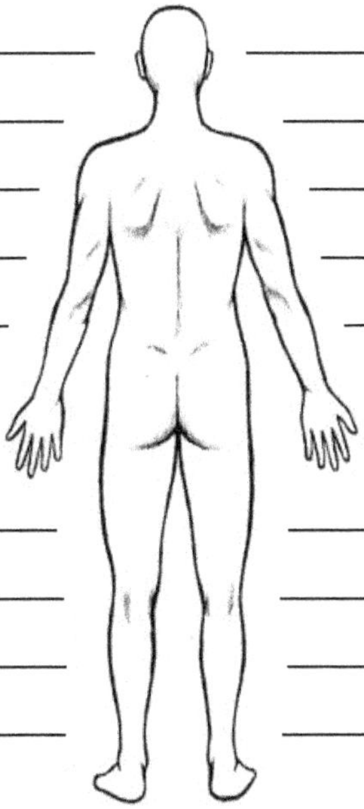

TRUST YOUR HEART ♥ TRUST YOUR HEART ♥

SHOULDERS: RESPONSIBILITY ♥ SHOULDERS: RESPONSIBILITY

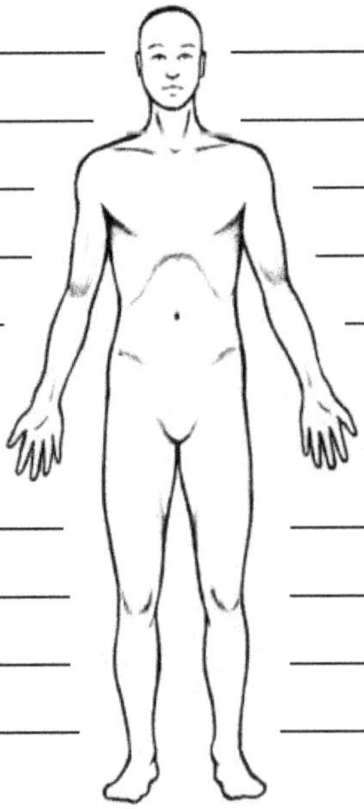

SHOULDERS: RESPONSIBILITY ♥ SHOULDERS: RESPONSIBILITY

SHOULDERS: RESPONSIBILITY ♥ SHOULDERS: RESPONSIBILITY

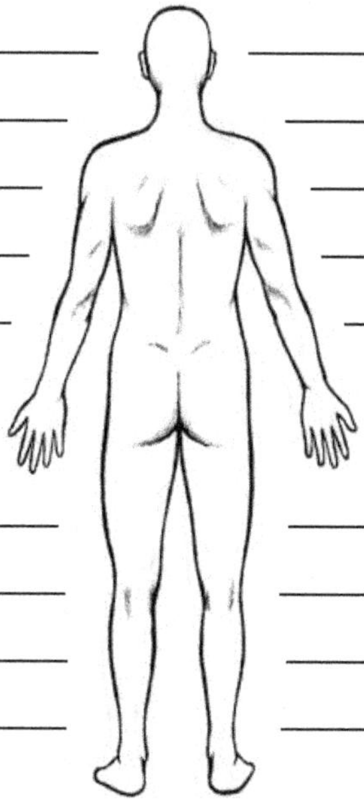

RESPONSE-ABILITY ♥ RESPONSE-ABILITY

RESPONSE-ABILITY ♥ RESPONSE-ABILITY

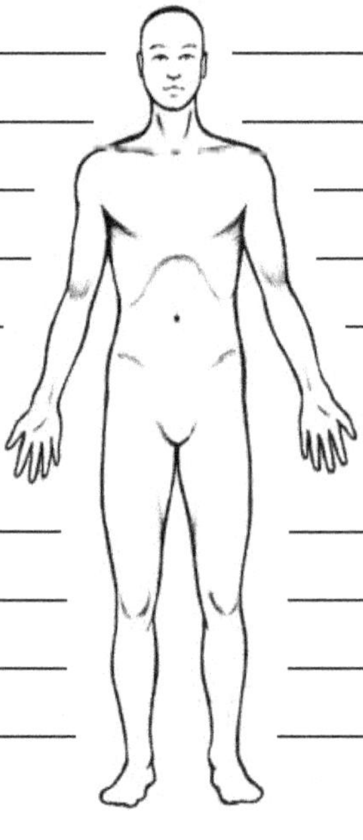

RESPONSE-ABILITY ♥ RESPONSE-ABILITY

RESPONSE-ABILITY ♥ RESPONSE-ABILITY

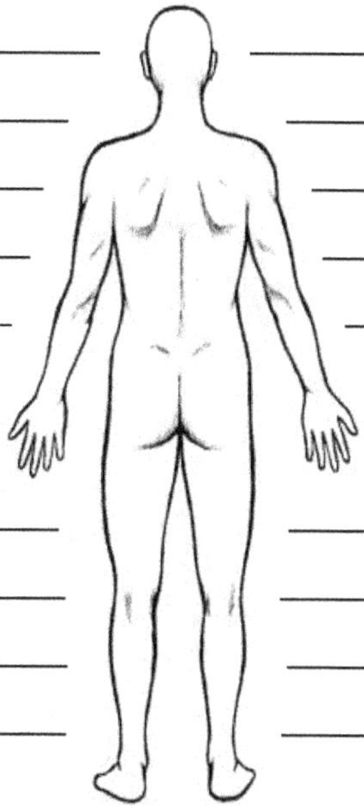

ARMS: EMBRACE ♥ ARMS: EMBRACE ♥ ARMS: EMBRACE

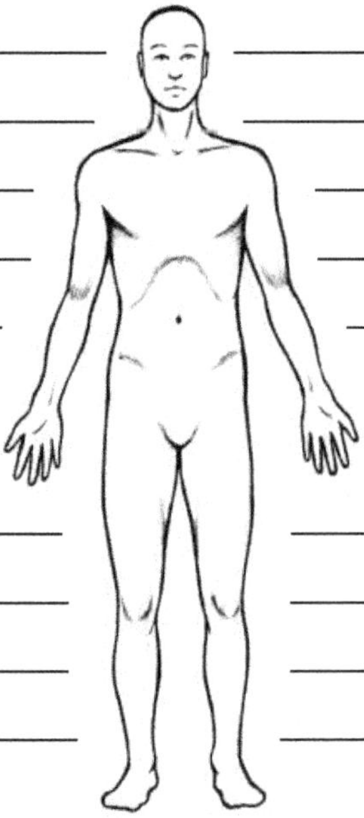

ARMS: EMBRACE ❤ ARMS: EMBRACE ❤ ARMS: EMBRACE

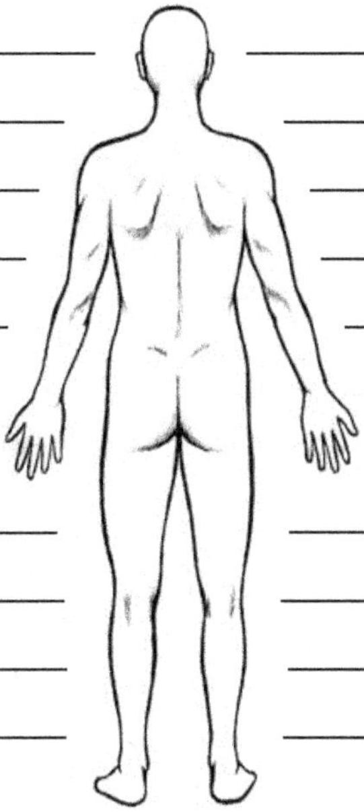

ARMS: EMBRACE ❤ ARMS: EMBRACE ❤

EMBRACE ALL THAT YOU FEEL ♥ EMBRACE ALL THAT YOU FEEL

EMBRACE ALL THAT YOU FEEL ♥ EMBRACE ALL THAT YOU FEEL

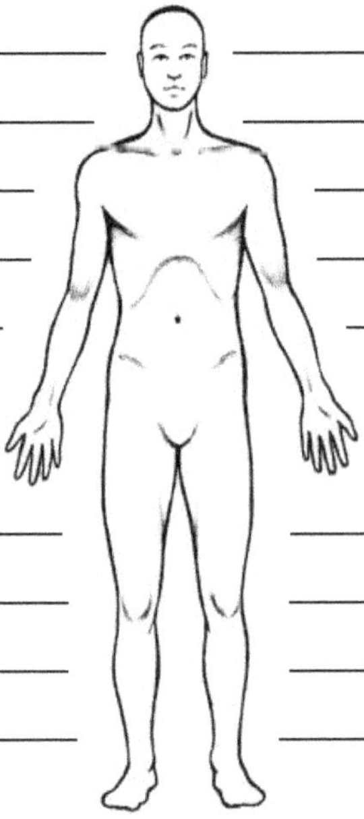

EMBRACE ALL THAT YOU FEEL ♥ EMBRACE ALL THAT YOU FEEL

EMBRACE ALL THAT YOU FEEL ♥ EMBRACE ALL THAT YOU FEEL ♥

EMBRACE ALL THAT YOU FEEL ♥ EMBRACE ALL THAT YOU FEEL

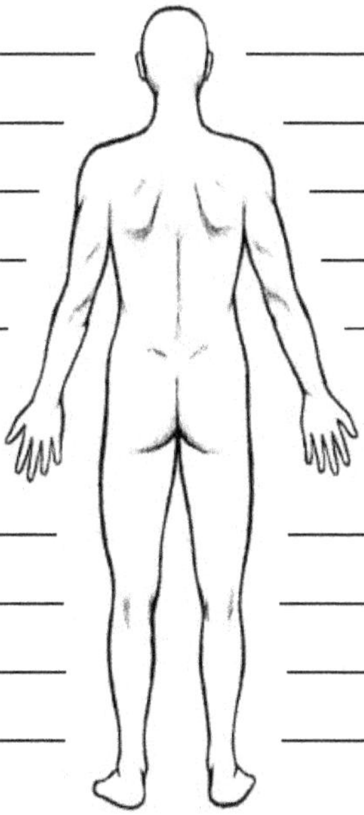

EMBRACE ALL THAT YOU FEEL ♥ EMBRACE ALL THAT YOU FEEL ♥

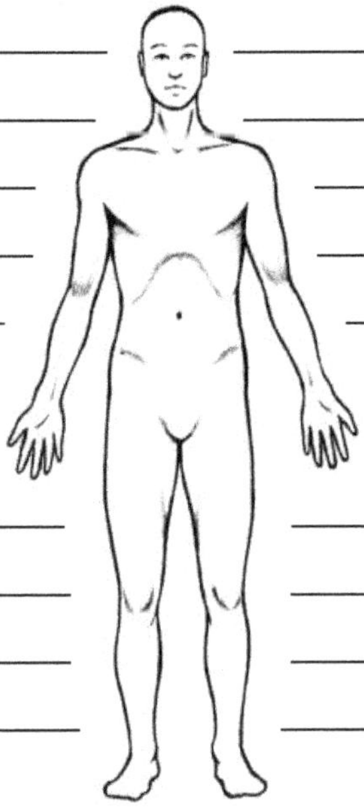

HANDS: GIVE & RECEIVE ♥ HANDS: GIVE & RECEIVE ♥ HANDS: GIVE & RECEIVE

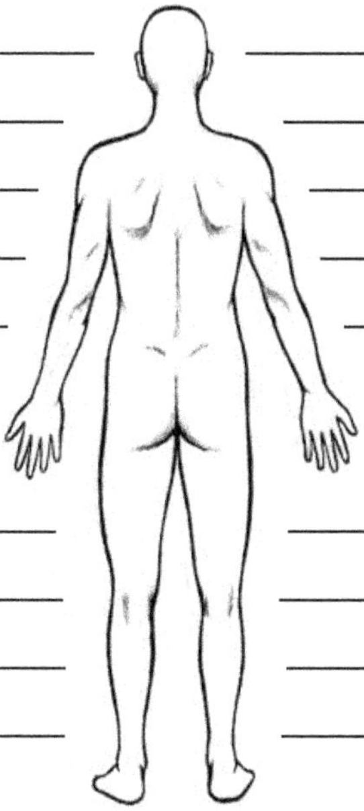

GIVING IS RECEIVING ♥ RECEIVING IS GIVING

RECEIVING IS GIVING

♥

GIVING IS RECEIVING

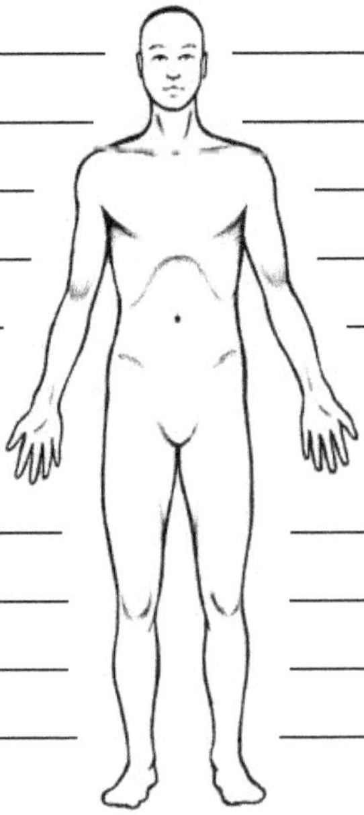

GIVING IS RECEIVING ♥ RECEIVING IS GIVING

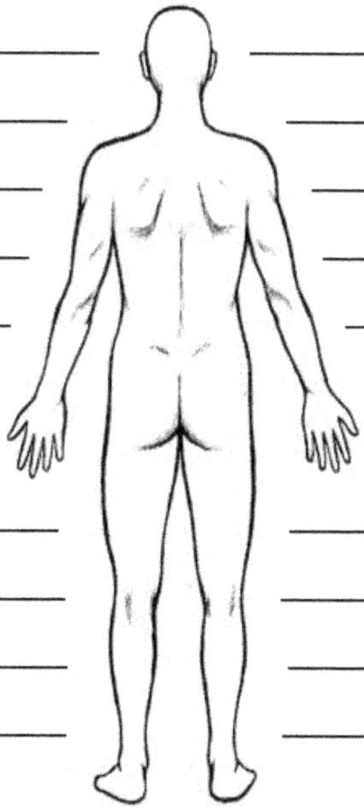

GIVING IS RECEIVING ♥ RECEIVING IS GIVING

NECK: PATH OF COMMUNICATION BETWEEN HEAD & HEART

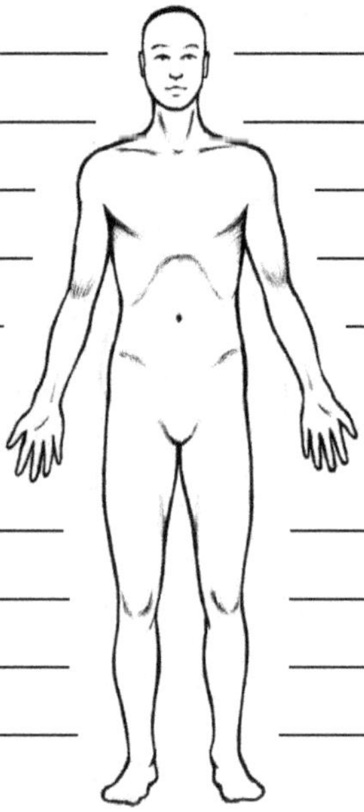

NECK: PATH OF COMMUNICATION BETWEEN HEAD & HEART

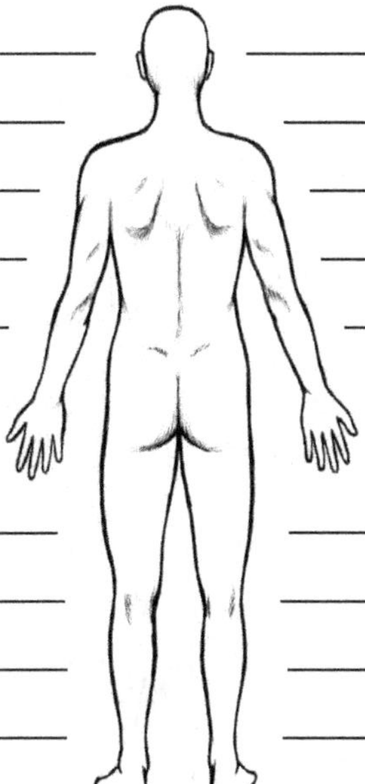

SPEAK THE WISDOM OF YOUR HEART ♥ SPEAK THE WISDOM OF YOUR HEART

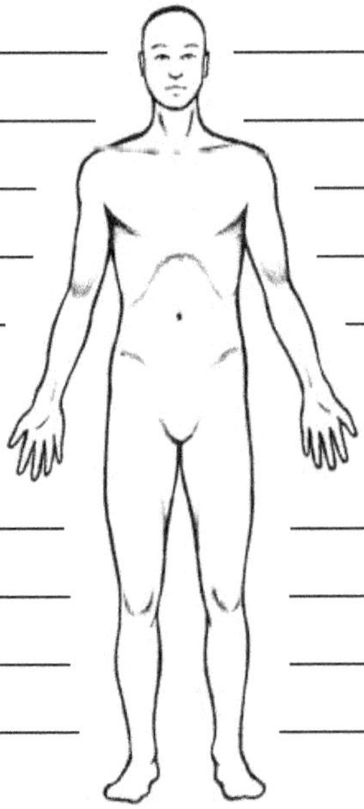

SPEAK THE WISDOM OF YOUR HEART ♥ SPEAK THE WISDOM OF YOUR HEART ♥

SPEAK THE WISDOM OF YOUR HEART ♥ SPEAK THE WISDOM OF YOUR HEART

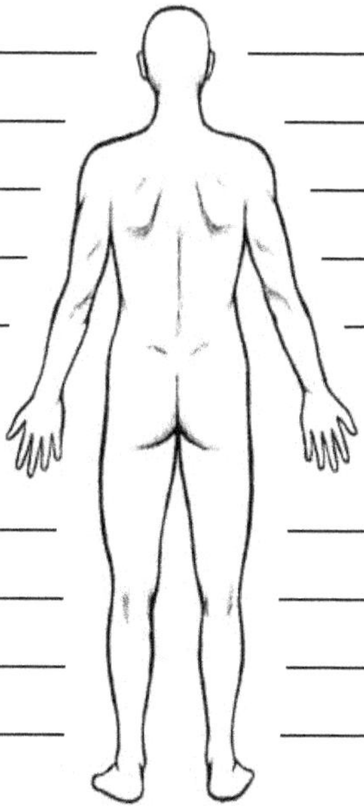

SPEAK THE WISDOM OF YOUR HEART ♥ SPEAK THE WISDOM OF YOUR HEART ♥

HEAD: WHERE YOU HOLD YOUR THOUGHTS ♥ HEAD: WHERE YOU HOLD YOUR THOUGHTS

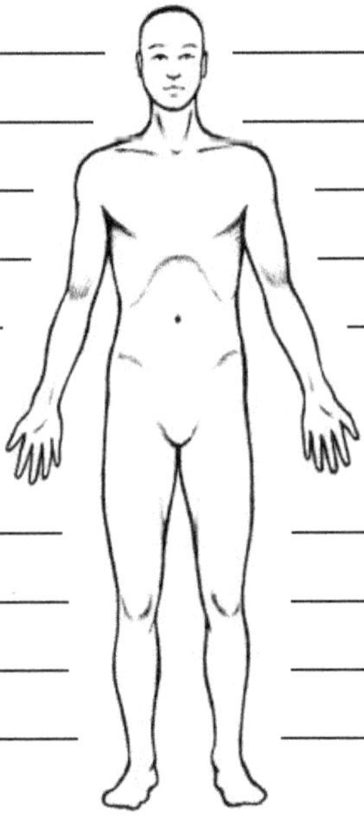

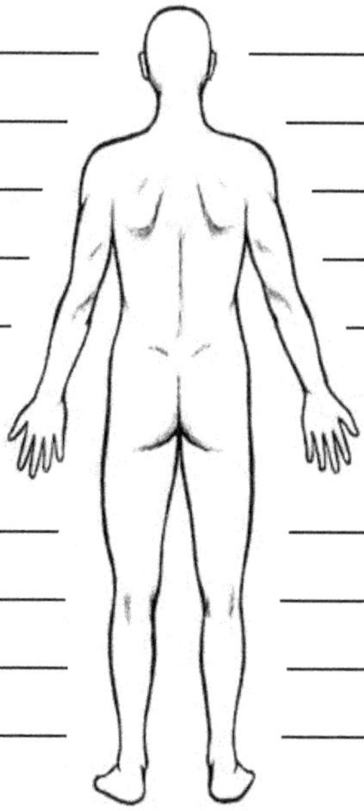

HEAD: WHERE YOU HOLD YOUR THOUGHTS ♥ HEAD: WHERE YOU HOLD YOUR THOUGHTS

KNOW YOUR WISDOM ♥ KNOW YOUR WISDOM ♥ KNOW YOUR WISDOM

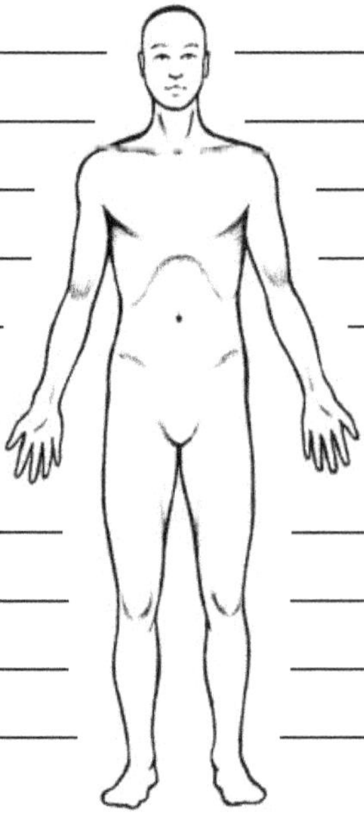

KNOW YOUR WISDOM ♥ KNOW YOUR WISDOM ♥ KNOW YOUR WISDOM

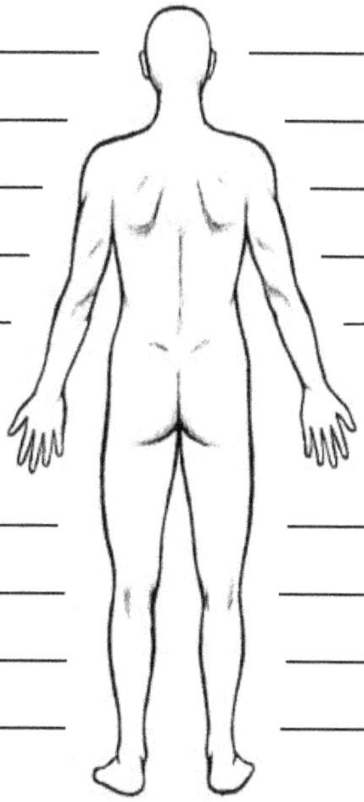

KNOW YOUR WISDOM ♥ KNOW YOUR WISDOM ♥

FACE: HOW YOU FACE THE WORLD ♥ FACE: HOW YOU FACE THE WORLD ♥ FACE: HOW YOU FACE THE WORLD

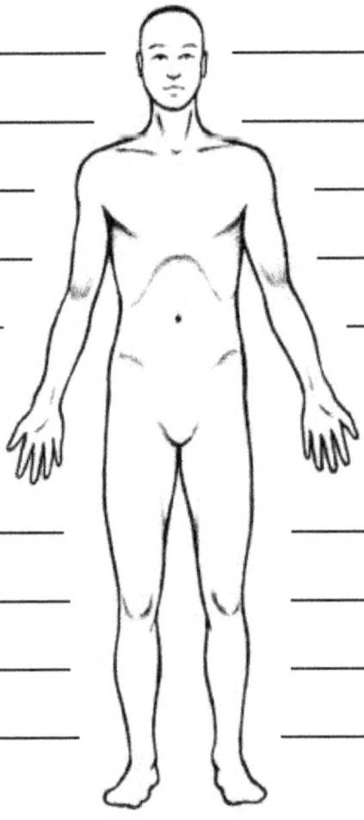

FACE: HOW YOU FACE THE WORLD ♥ FACE: HOW YOU FACE THE WORLD

FACE: HOW YOU FACE THE WORLD ♥ FACE: HOW YOU FACE THE WORLD ♥ FACE: HOW YOU FACE THE WORLD

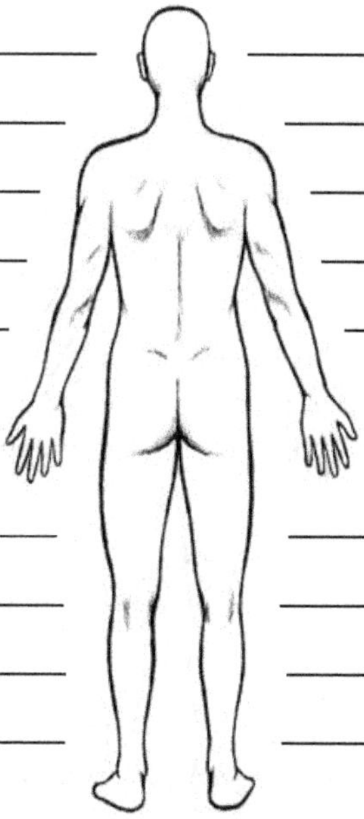

FACE THE WORLD FROM WITHIN ♥ FACE THE WORLD FROM WITHIN

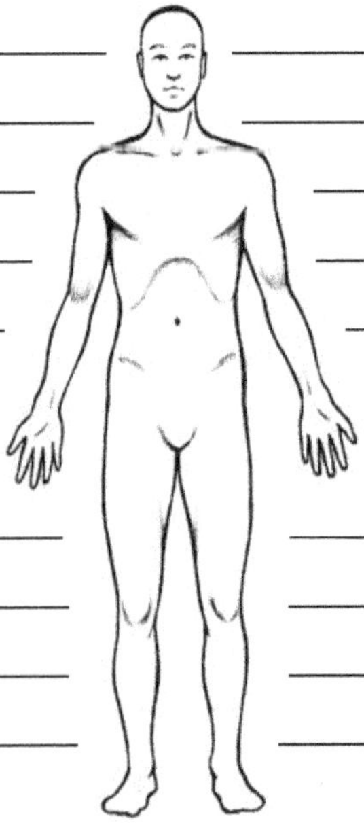

FACE THE WORLD FROM WITHIN ♥ FACE THE WORLD FROM WITHIN

FACE THE WORLD FROM WITHIN ♥ FACE THE WORLD FROM WITHIN ♥

FACE THE WORLD FROM WITHIN ♥ FACE THE WORLD FROM WITHIN

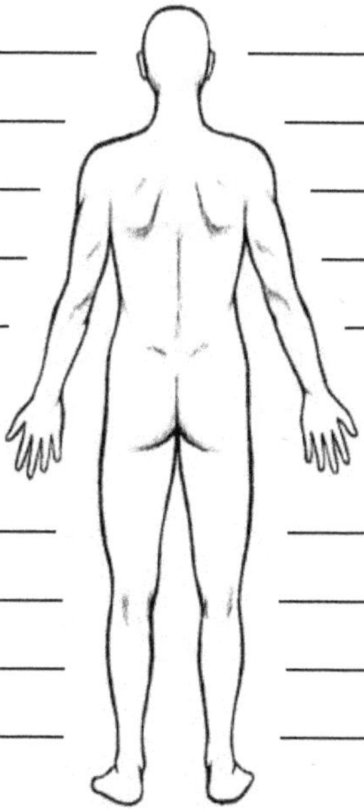

FACE THE WORLD FROM WITHIN ♥ FACE THE WORLD FROM WITHIN ♥

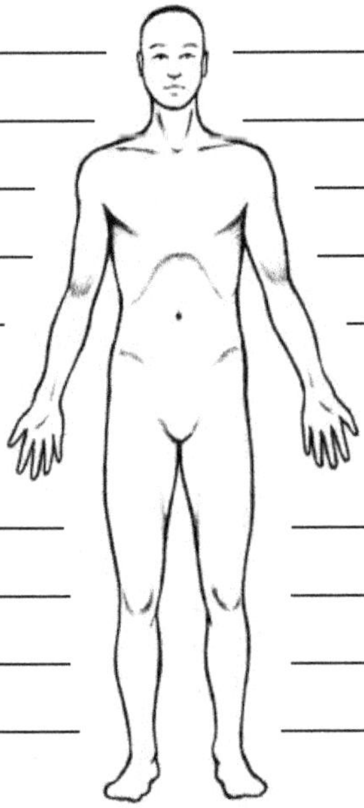

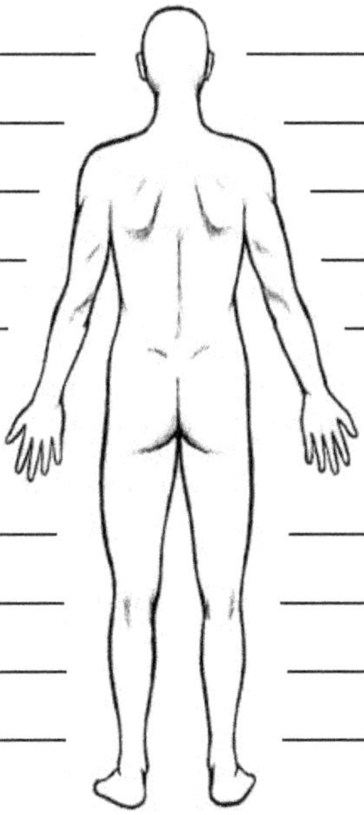

Doreen Rivera has been called the Godmother of Stretch. Doreen introduced stretch to Jane Fonda, and through her affiliation with Jane Fonda's Workout, stretch class has become a staple in the exercise world we know today. She has taught her program at UCLA Department of Biological Sciences Extension Division and Dr. Leroy Perry's International Sportscience Institute. She was Health Editor for the original Latina magazine. She was on the Board of Directors for Femmy DeLyser's ground-breaking pregnancy program. Doreen also served as John Travolta's stretch coach for his role in *Saturday Night Fever*. Her video, *Stretch For Life*, was reviewed by Shape magazine as the # 1 stretch video in the United States and Canada and was recommended in Cher's book, *Forever Fit*. Doreen hosted her own exercise cable show, *RSVP*, in Los Angeles. Her work is the inspiration for many exercise programs, videos and books.

Doreen continues to teach this life-changing work through movement classes, workshops, seminars, individual sessions and her pregnancy program.

Doreen is currently bringing The Bodyful Mind® to the Los Angeles Unified School District curriculum by helping children develop emotional intelligence through movement and experiential dialogue. The Bodyful Mind Process® is geared toward evolving the emotional intelligence of every phase and each experience of life - from birth to death and everything in between.

Doreen Rivera's
The Bodyful Mind Institute
www.drbmi.com
info@drbmi.com

♥

Acknowledgements

Figure Illustration:
Alison Daddo & Scott Ramirez
for the gift that comes from their hands.

♥

Cover Illustration and Design:
Andy Candelaria, Candelaria Advertising
for capturing my vision so beautifully.

♥

Susan Grace,
Managing Director
for keeping the love light burnng.

♥

Published by Bodyful Mind Press
Published April 2012
2nd Edition
First Published December 2008

www.ingramcontent.com/pod-product-compliance
Lightning Source LLC
Chambersburg PA
CBHW081147270326
41930CB00014B/3073
* 9 7 8 0 9 8 2 2 4 3 9 0 9 *